Science Stories of Ancient China

Distinguished Doctors of Ancient China

Written by Zhu Kang
Illustrated by Hong Tao and Feng Congying

Bian Que's Four Methods of Diagnosis
Hua Tuo's *Mafeisan* **and Five-Animal Exercises**
Wang Weiyi's Bronze Figure Inscribed with the Acupoints
Compendium of Materia Medica **by Li Shizhen**

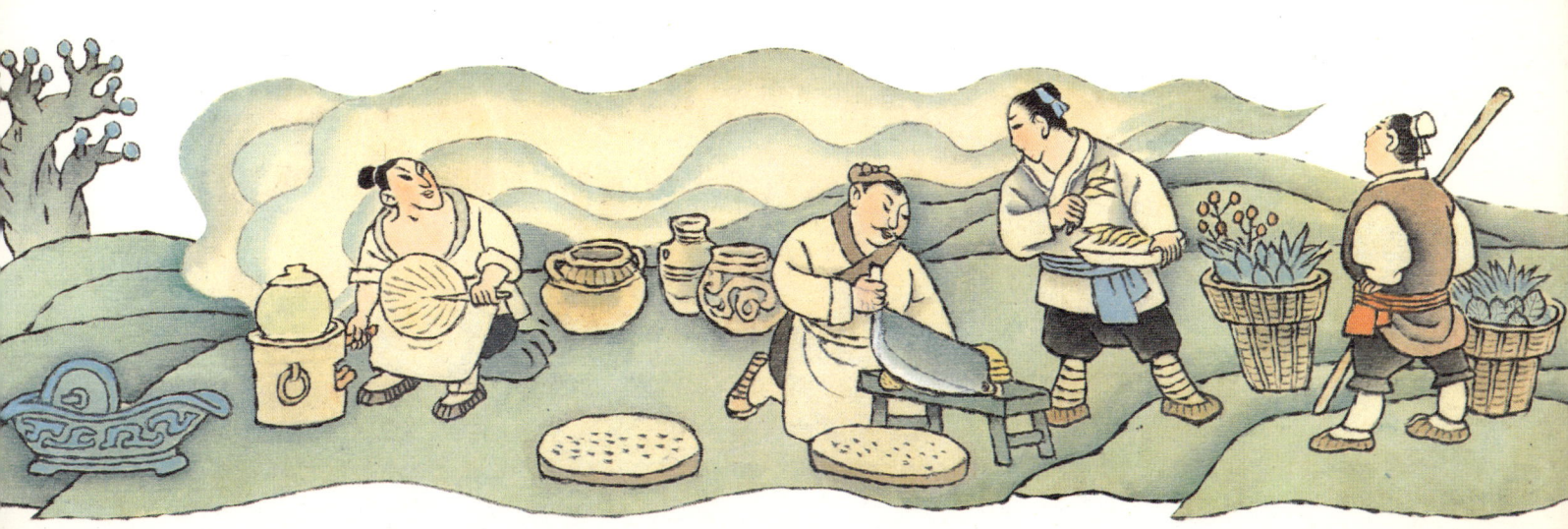

DOLPHIN BOOKS   BEIJING

First Edition 1996

ISBN 7-80051-870-1

© Dolphin Books, Beijing, 1996

Published by Dolphin Books
24 Baiwanzhuang Road, Beijing 100037, China

Distributed by China International Book Trading Corporation
35 Chegongzhuang Xilu, Beijing 100044, China
P.O. Box 399, Beijing, China

Printed in the People's Republic of China

Bian Que

Bian Que, originally named Qin Yueren (401-314 B.C.), was one of the founders of traditional Chinese medicine. It was he who first used and systematized traditional Chinese medical ways into the Four Methods of Diagnosis; that is, to observe, to smell, to ask and to feel.

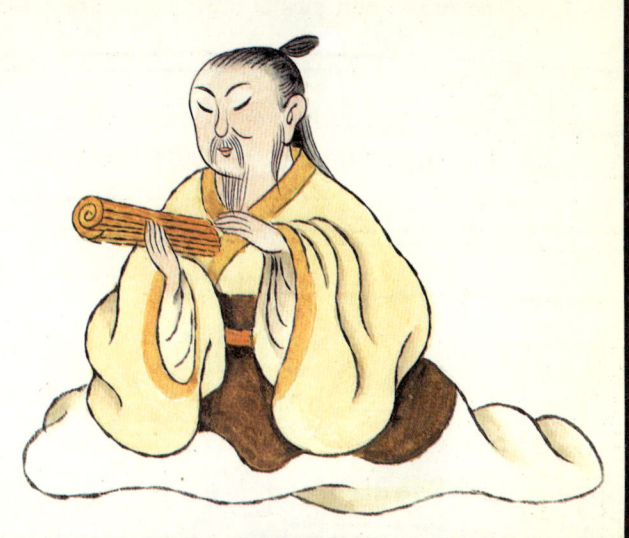

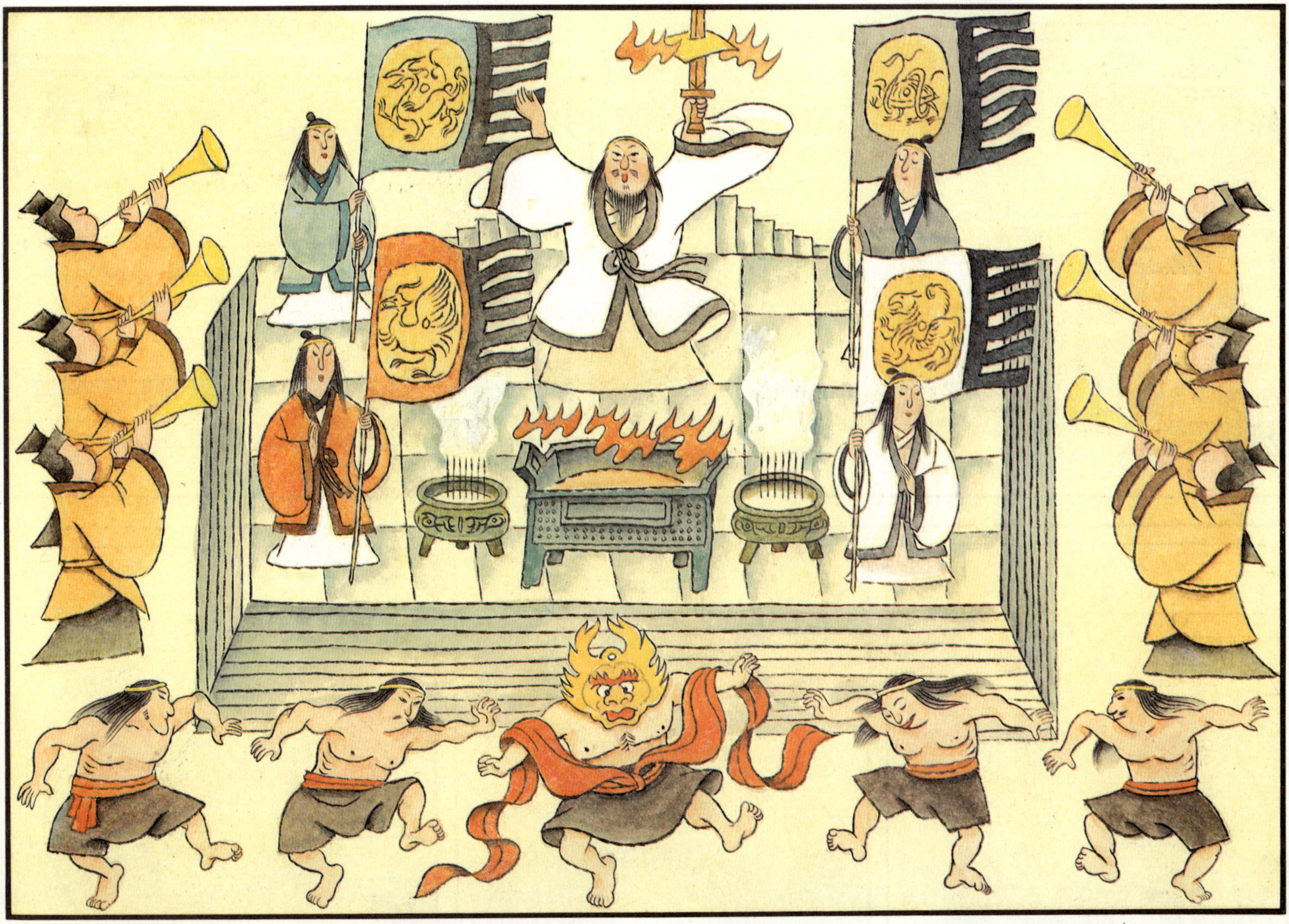

At that time, people attached more importance to ghosts and gods than to doctors. Whenever fatal epidemic diseases occurred, grand-scale ceremonies for getting rid of them were held and people prayed to the gods for soundness and safety.

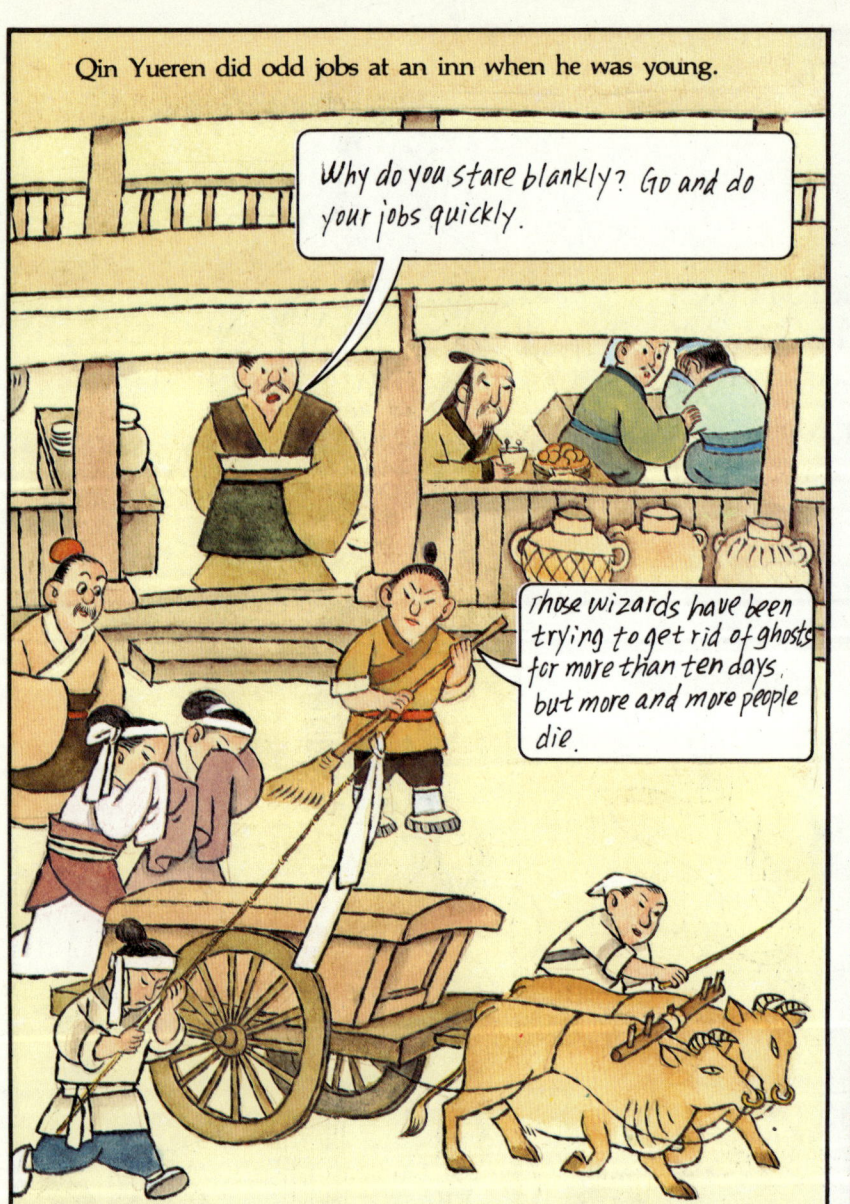
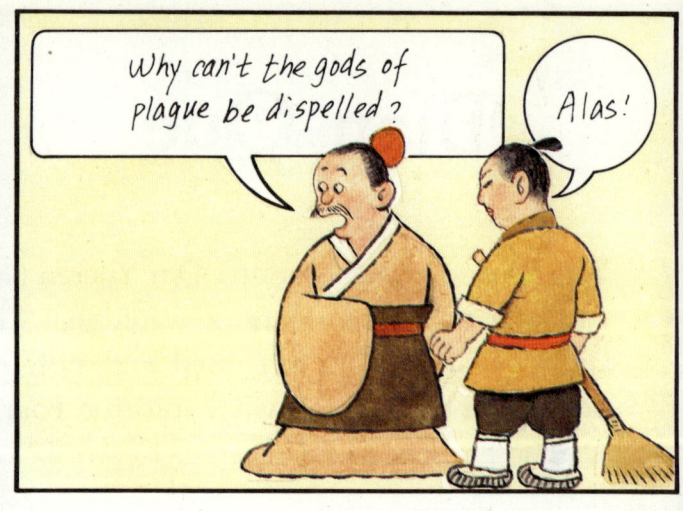
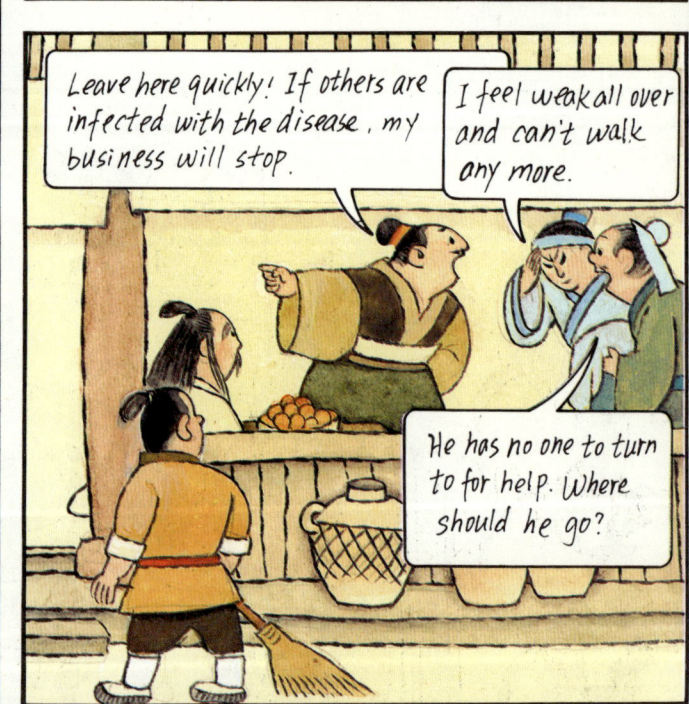
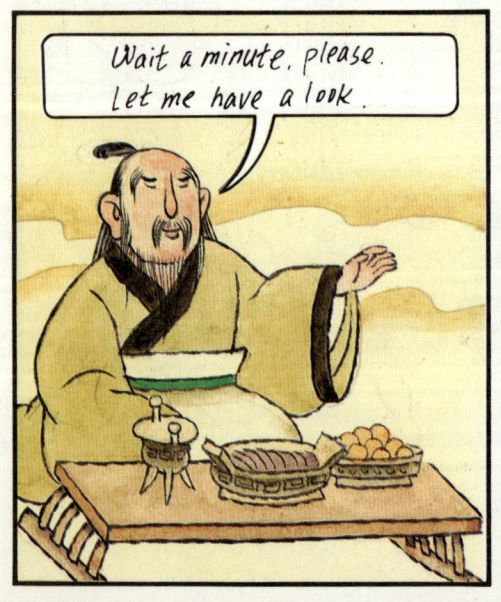
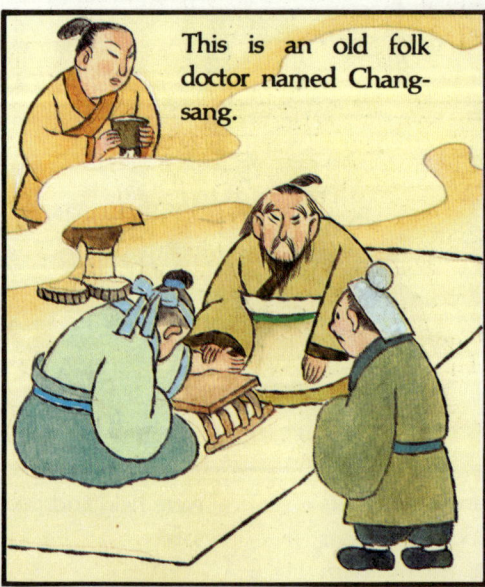
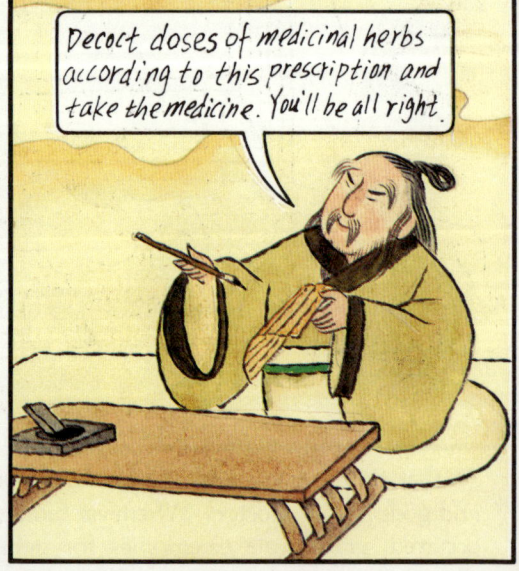

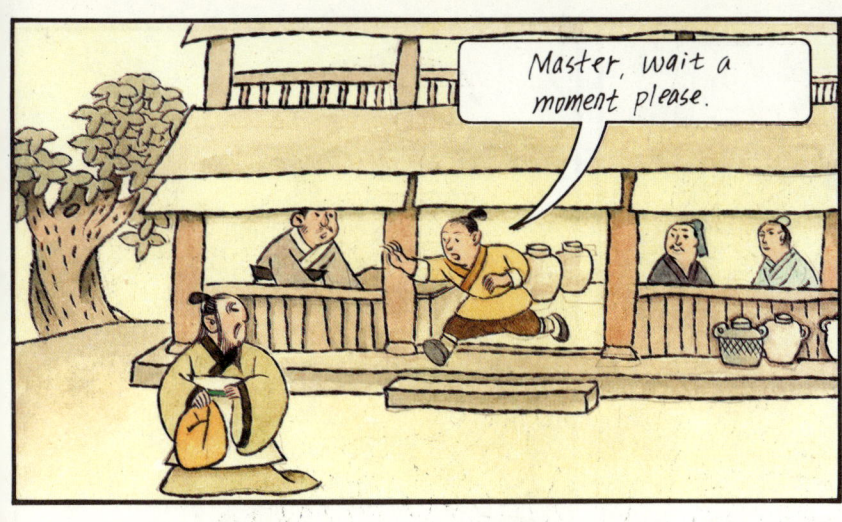
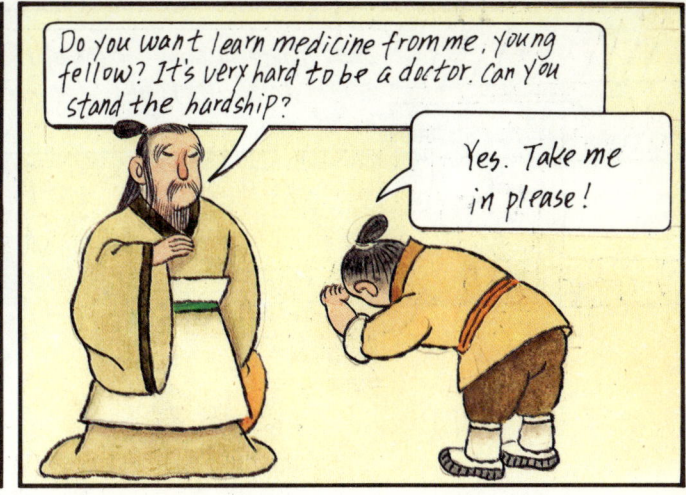

Qin Yueren began learning medicine.

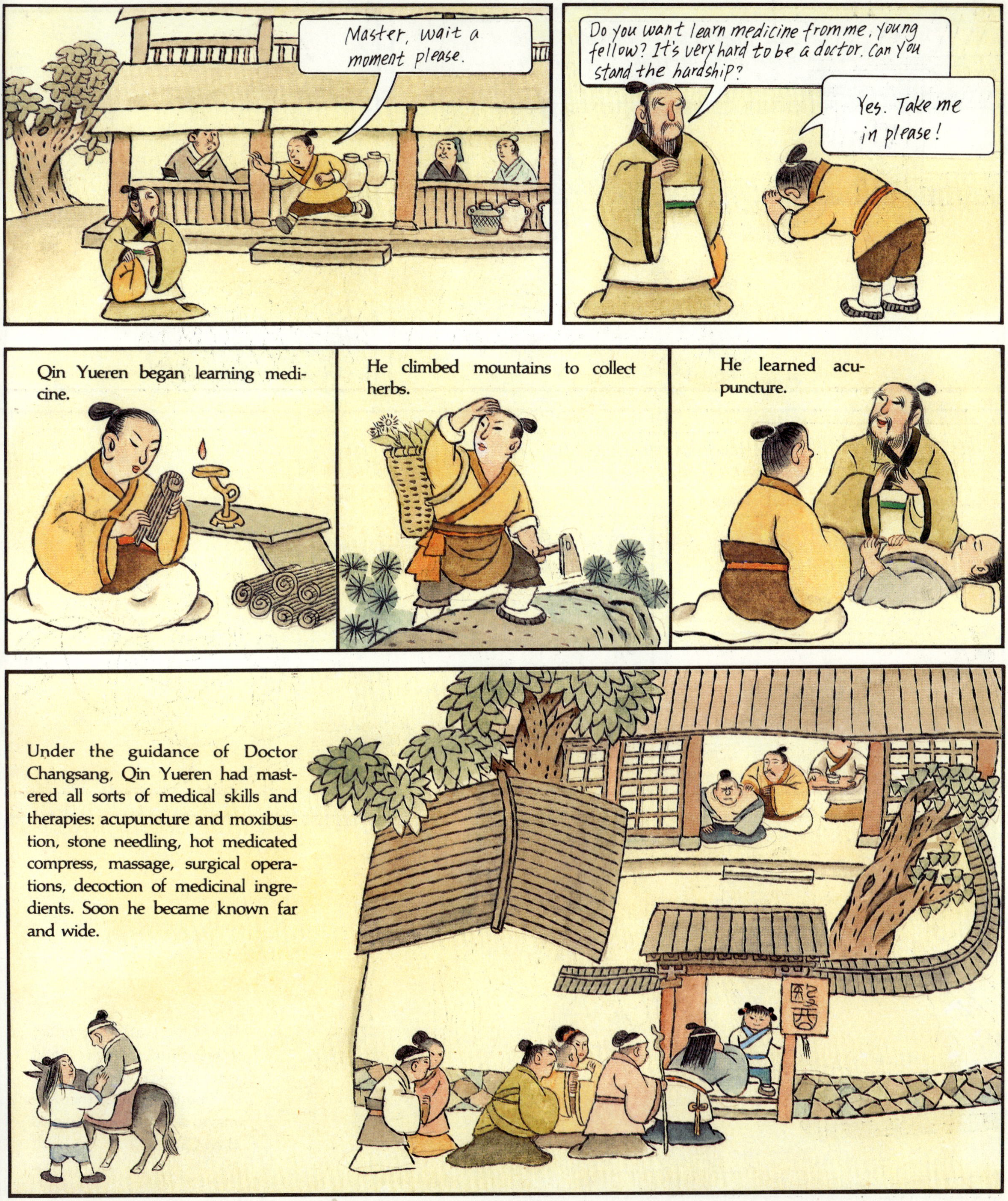

He climbed mountains to collect herbs.

He learned acupuncture.

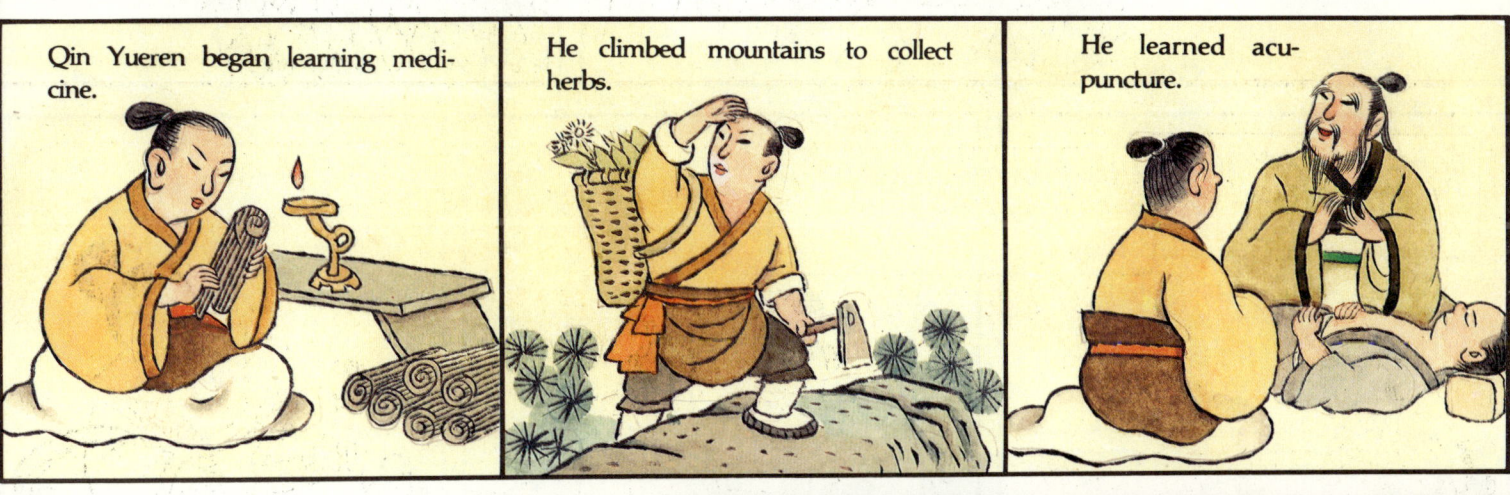

Under the guidance of Doctor Changsang, Qin Yueren had mastered all sorts of medical skills and therapies: acupuncture and moxibustion, stone needling, hot medicated compress, massage, surgical operations, decoction of medicinal ingredients. Soon he became known far and wide.

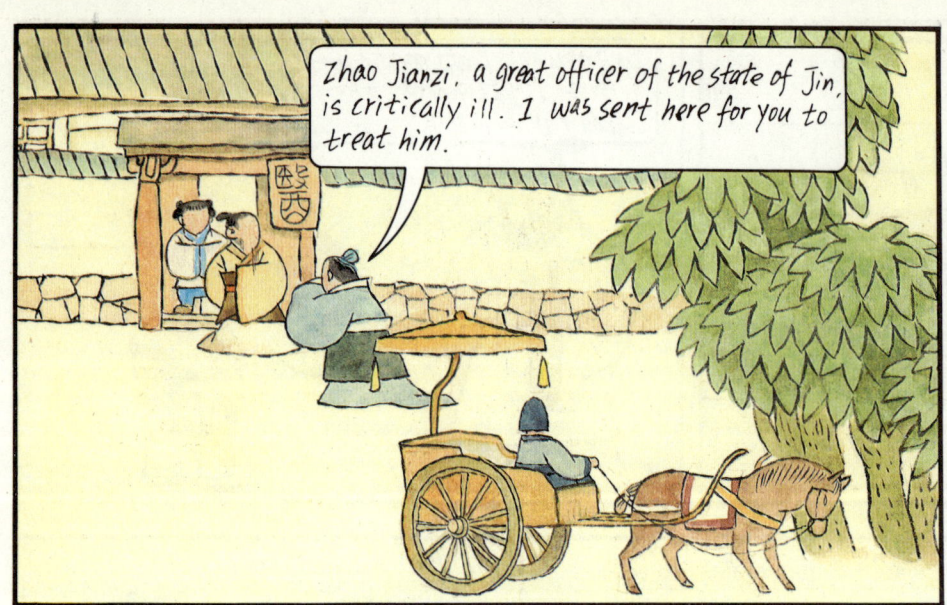
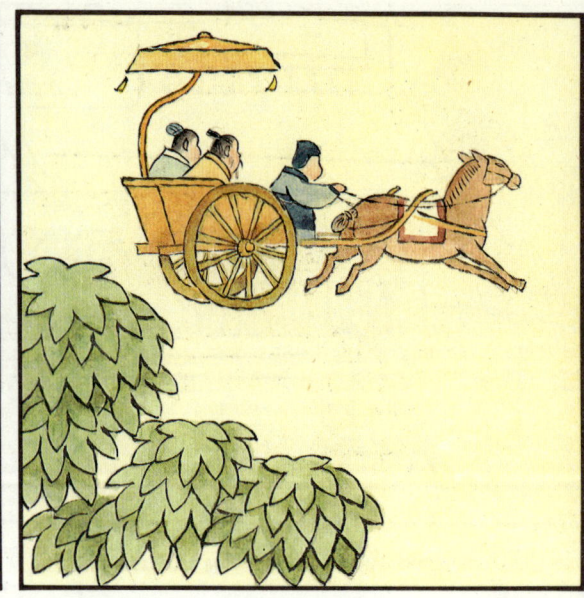
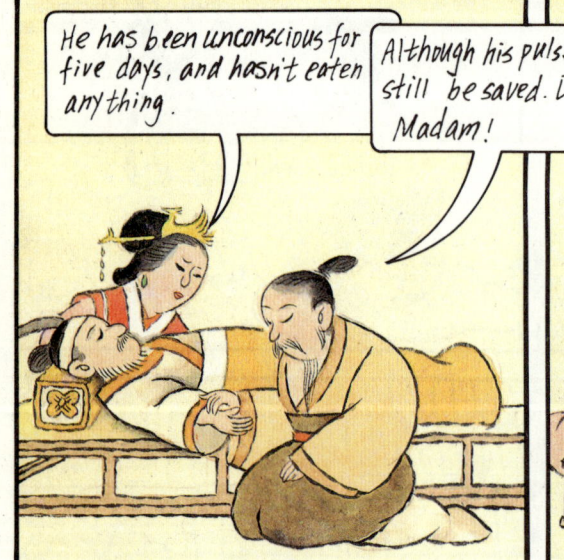
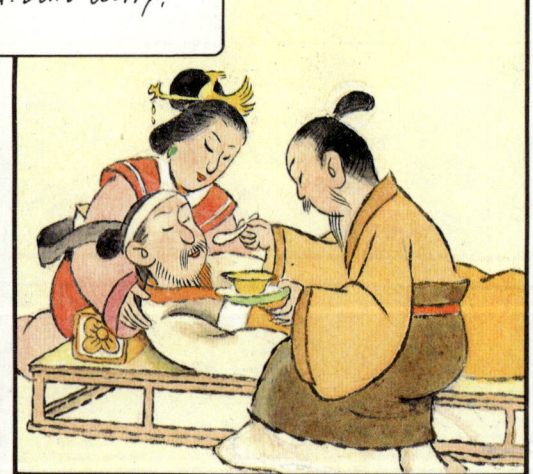
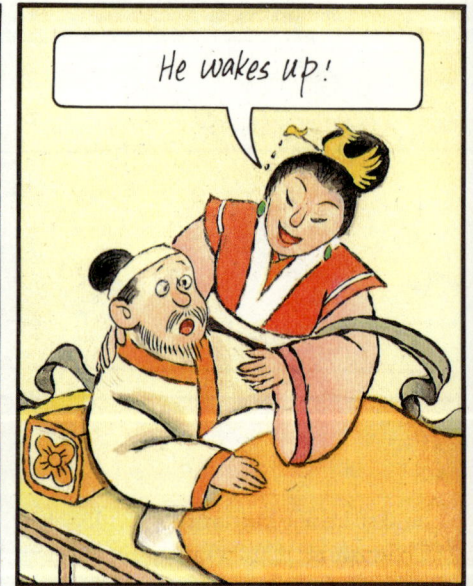
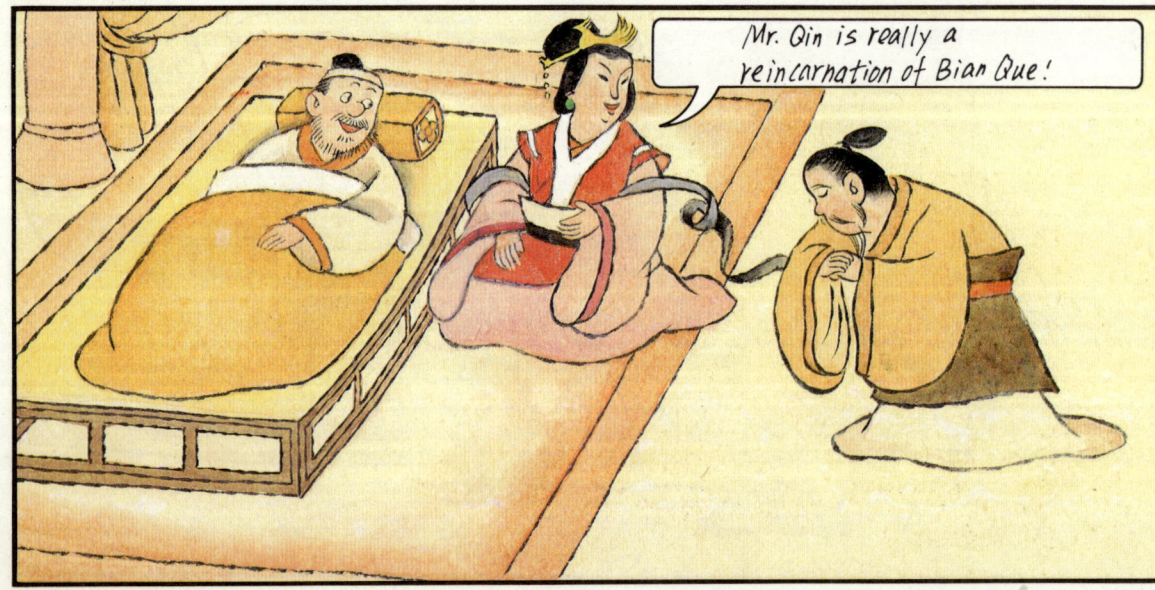

Bian Que was a legendary magic bird, which could cure people's diseases with its long beak. Since then the magic doctor was known as Bian Que.

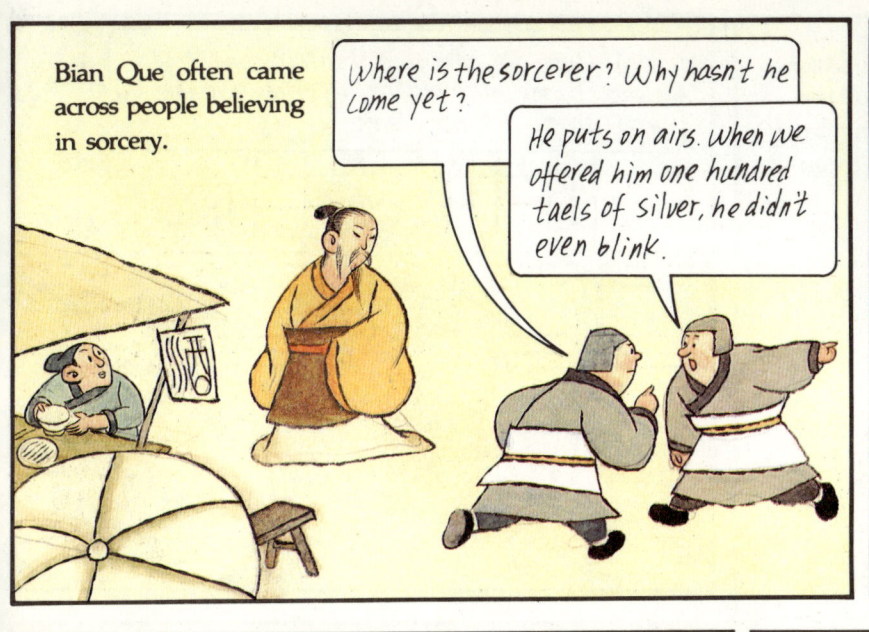

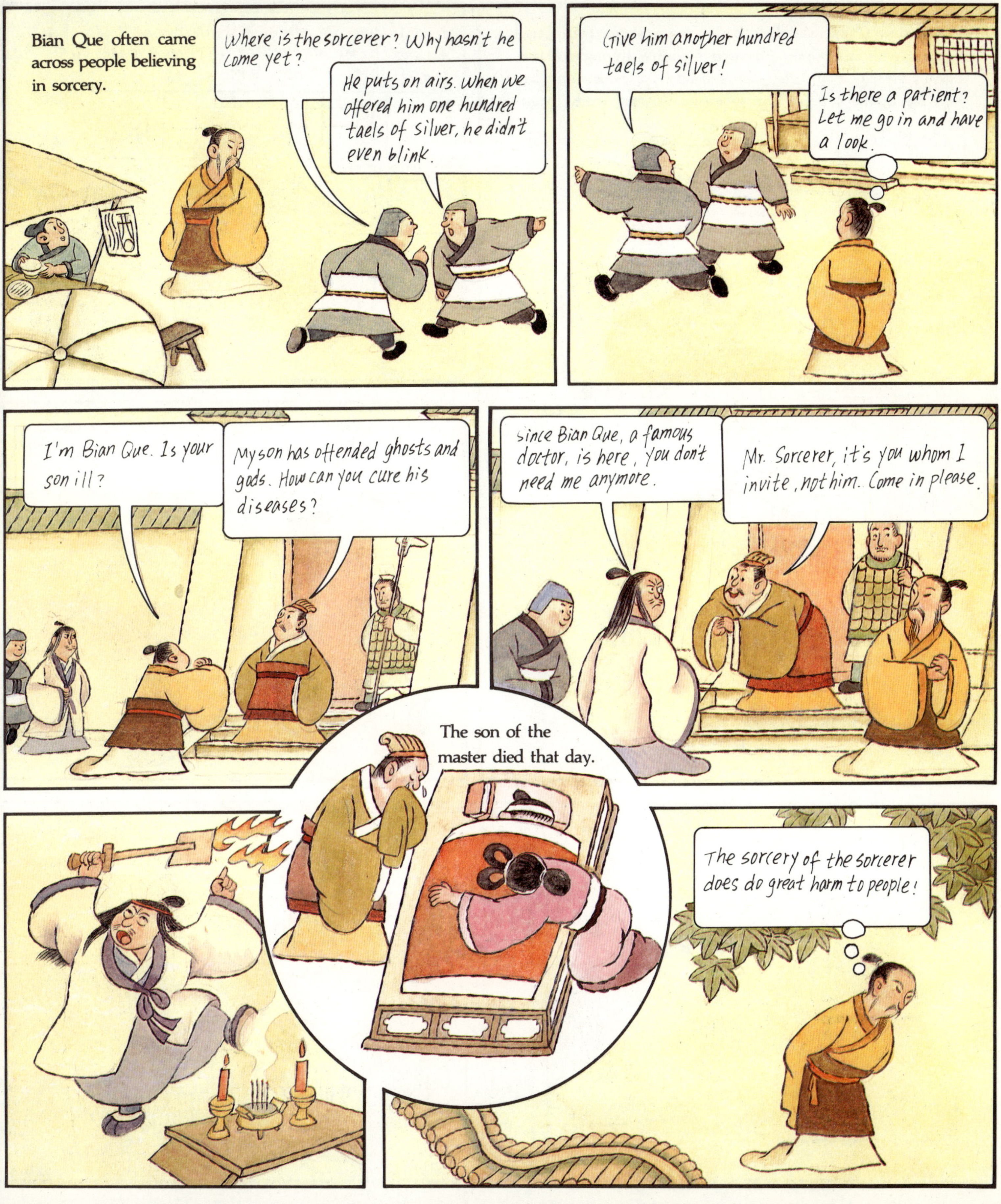

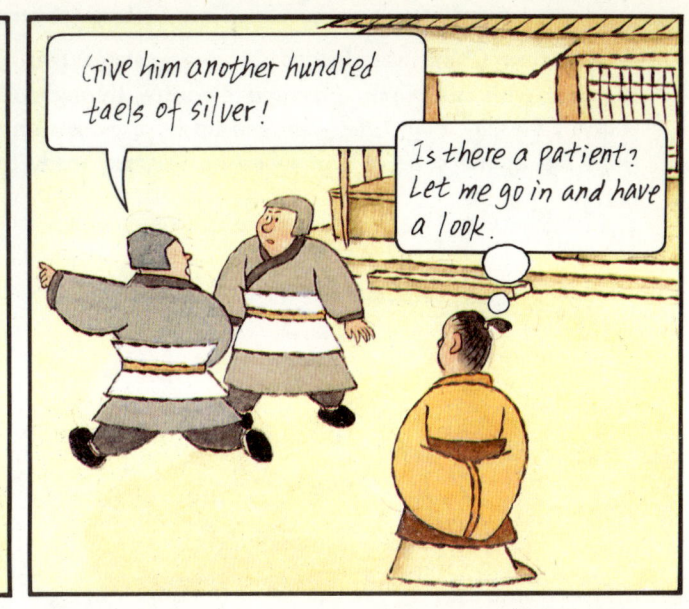

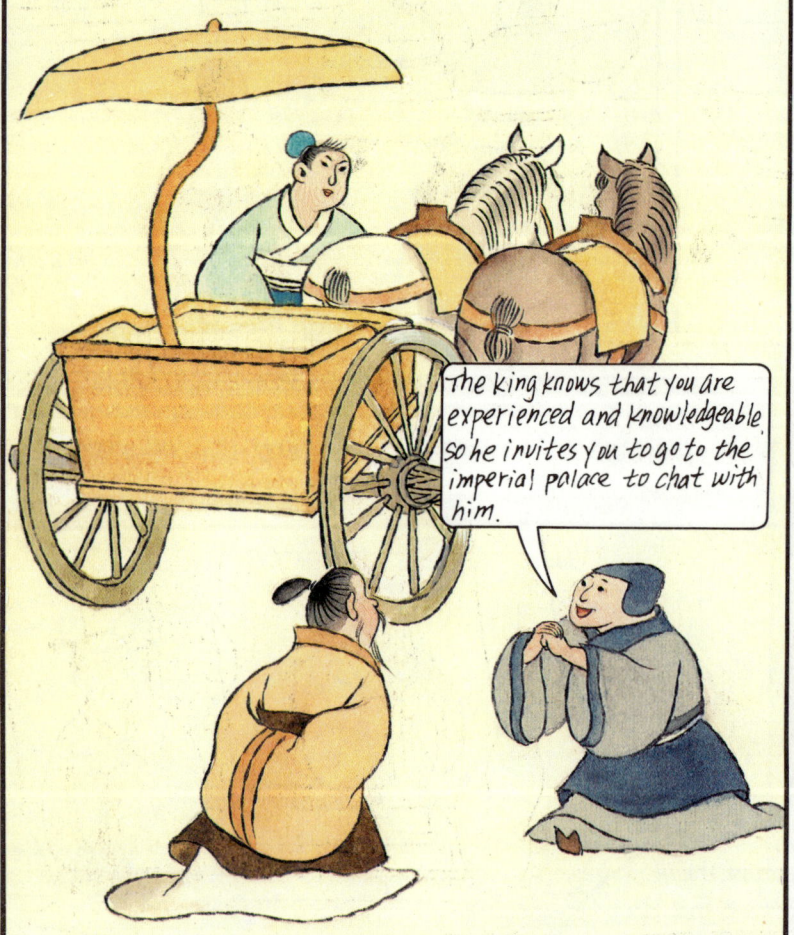

At that time China was divided into many states. Bian Que, together with his pupils, practised medicine throughout the states. One day Bian Que was held up by a person sent by the King of the state of Qin when he was just ready to go out.

The king knows that you are experienced and knowledgeable, so he invites you to go to the imperial palace to chat with him.

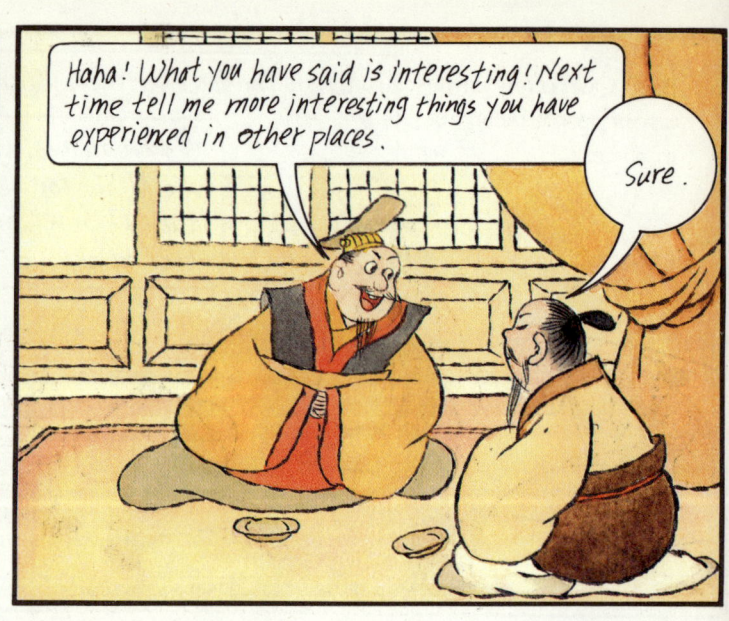

Haha! What you have said is interesting! Next time tell me more interesting things you have experienced in other places.

Sure.

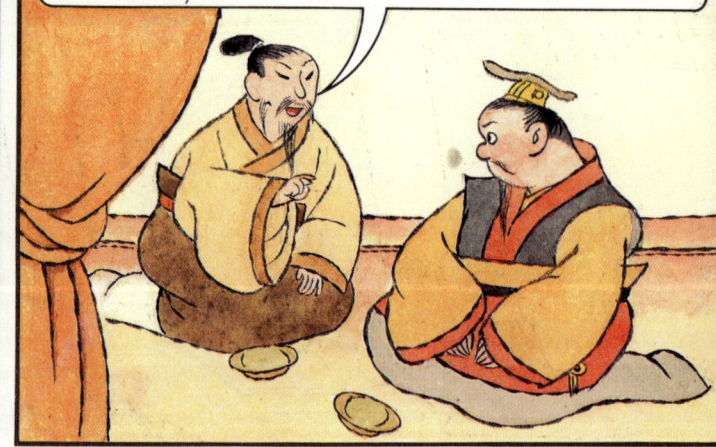

To speak frankly, Your Majesty, you have got a disease which is hidden inside your skin, and it should be treated immediately.

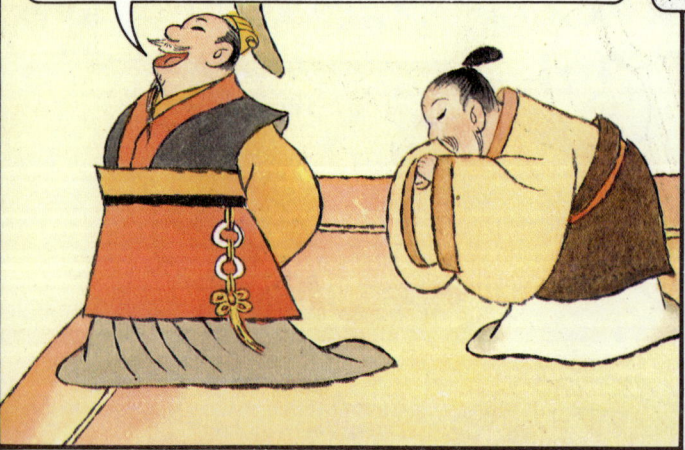

Have I got a disease? Inside the skin? Haha! You're making fun of me? Come on, see the doctor off!

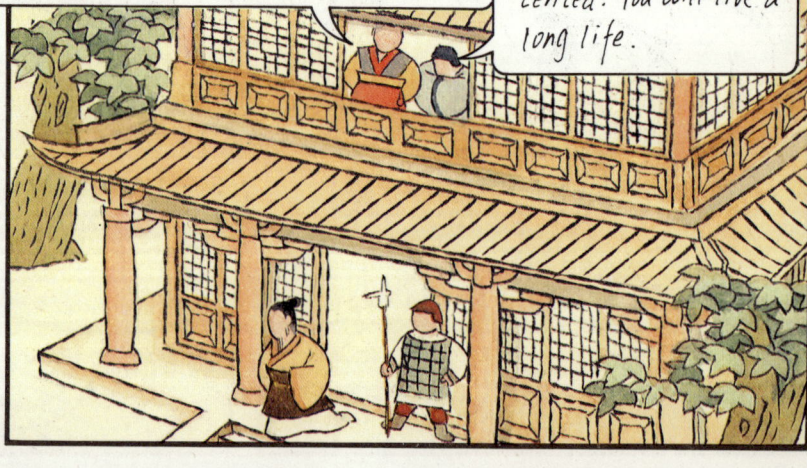

Doctors like to consider a healthy person a patient to show off their skills. Bian Que is a man like this!

Your Majesty is in high spirits, carefree and contented. You will live a long life.

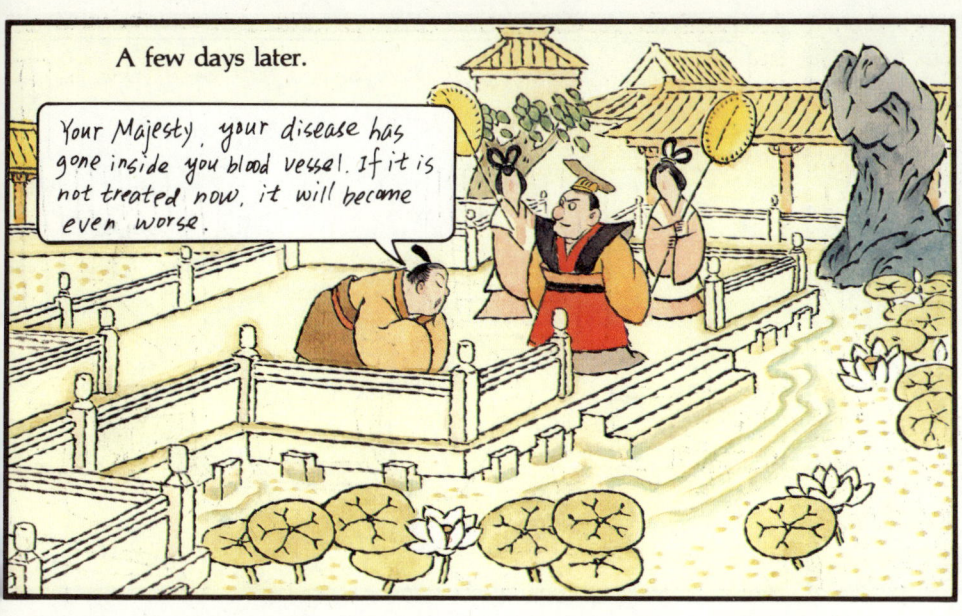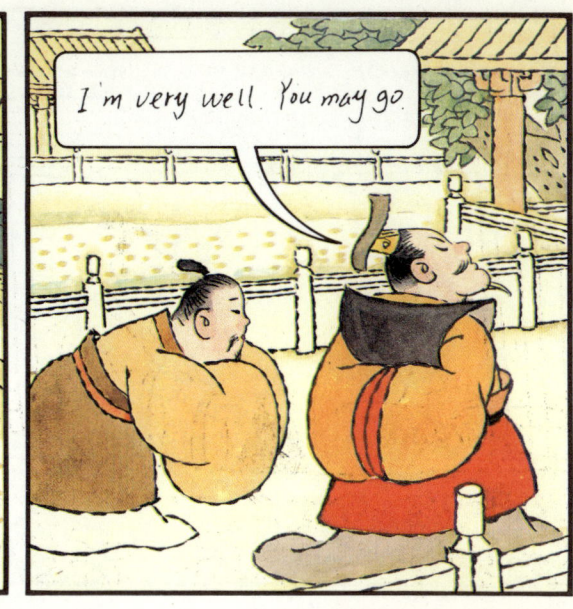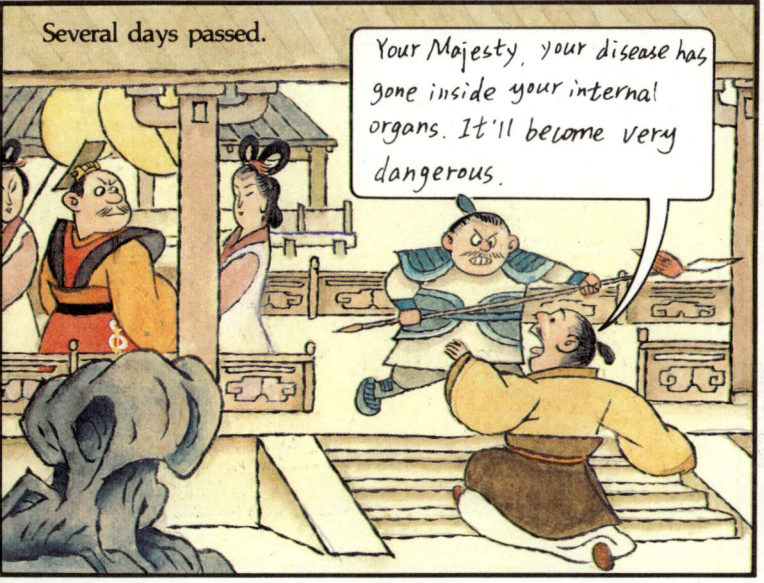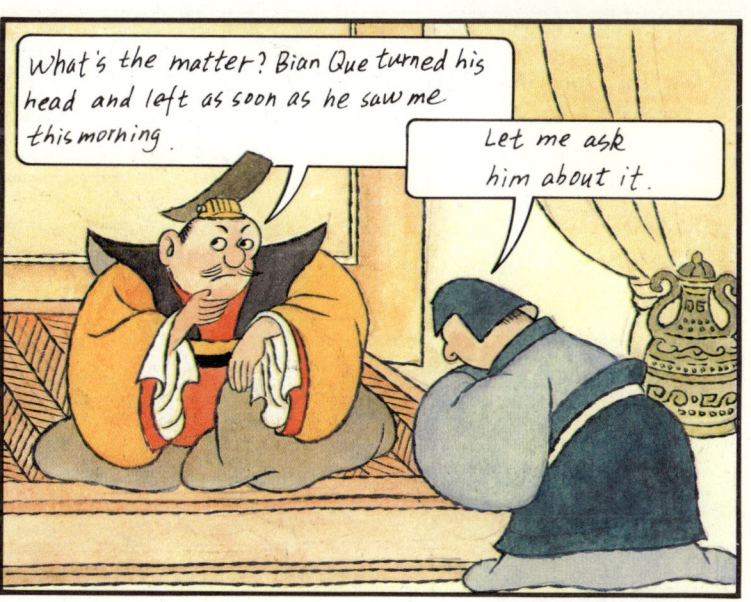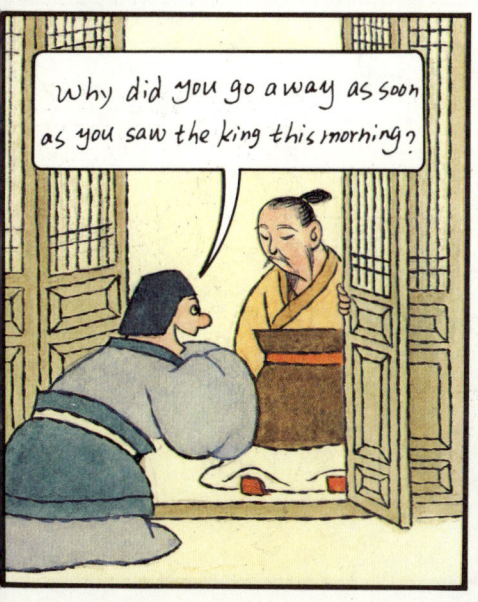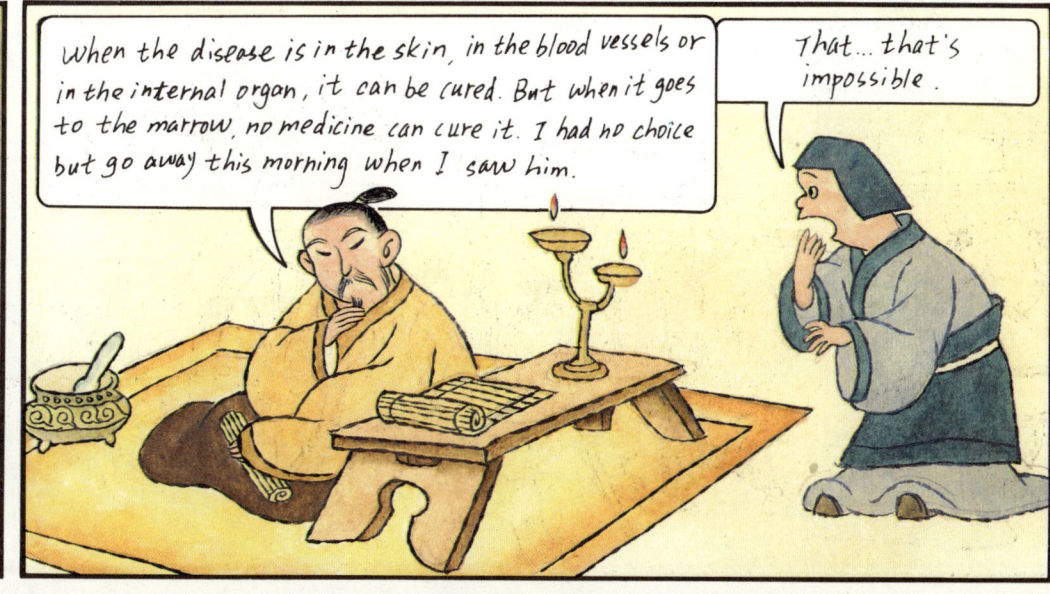

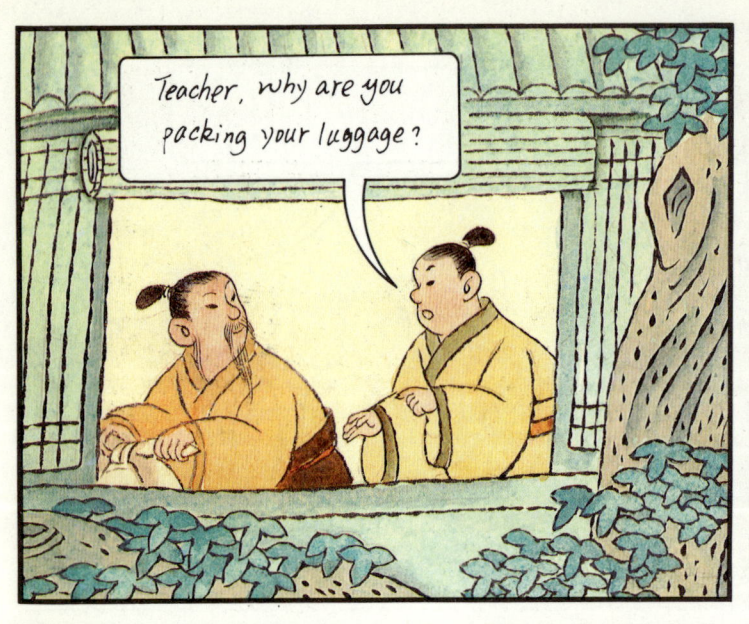
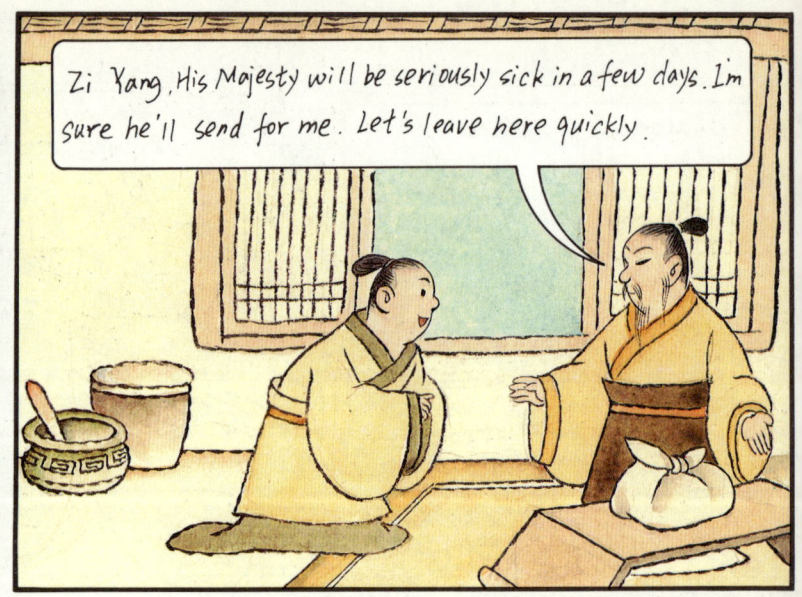
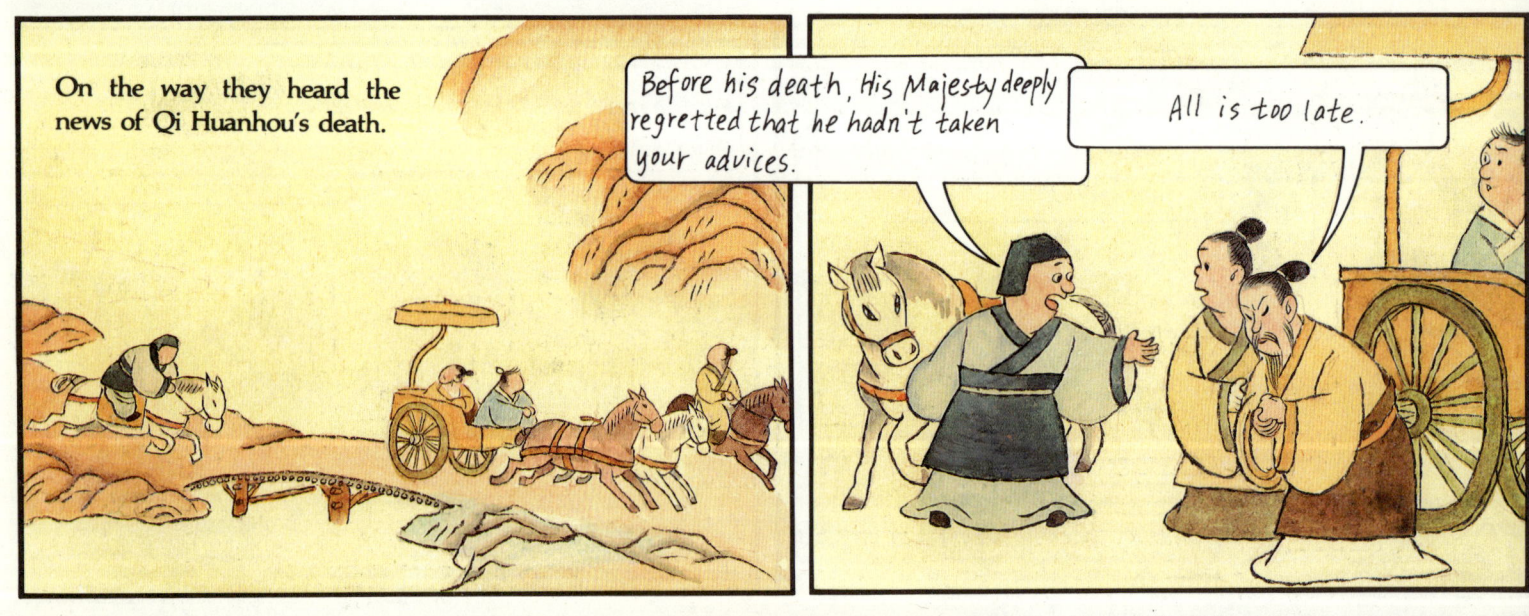
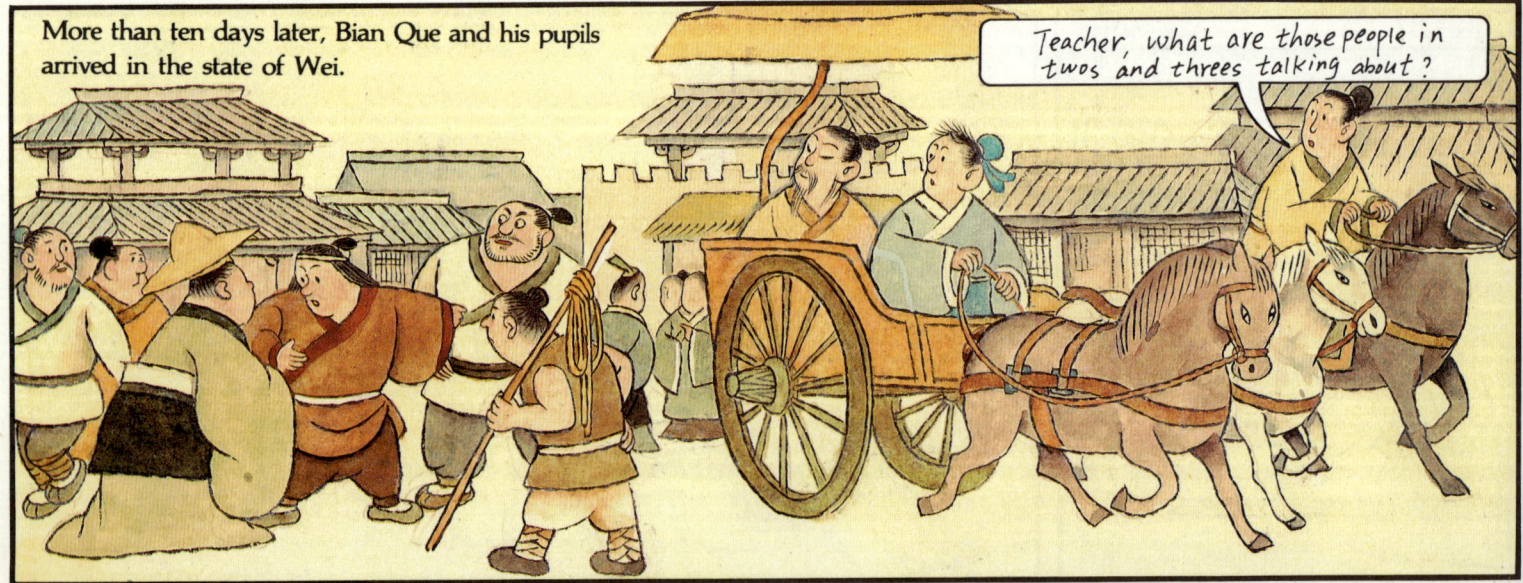

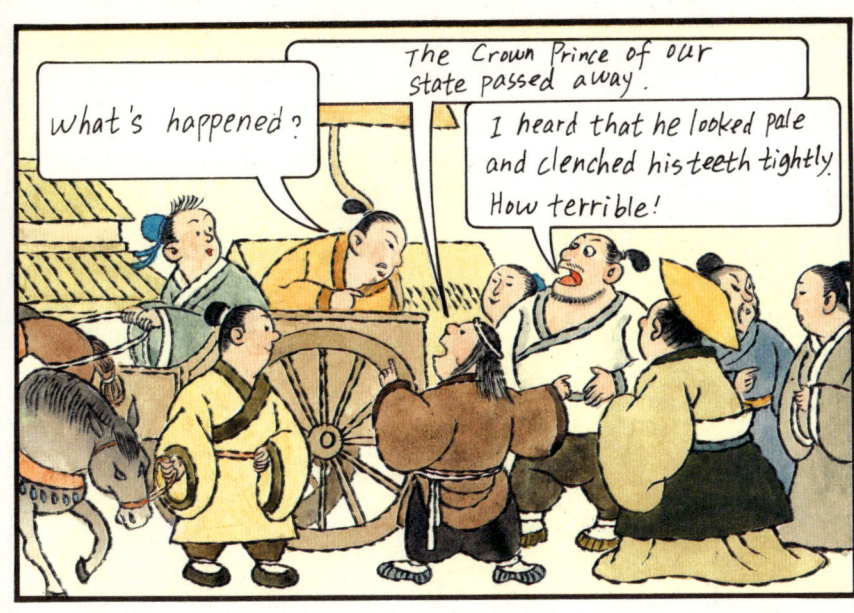
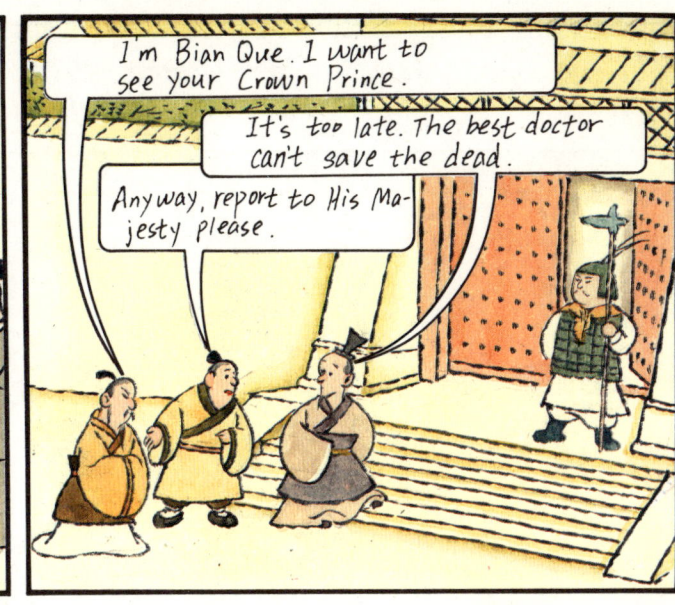
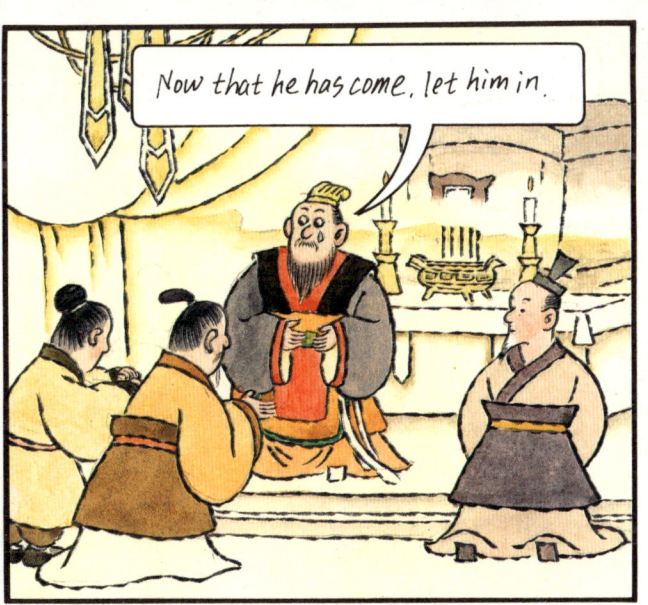
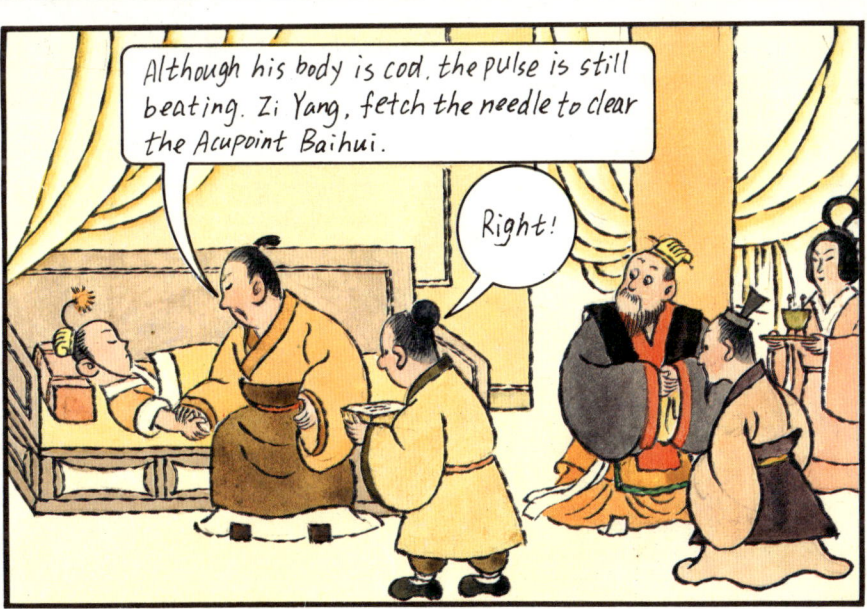
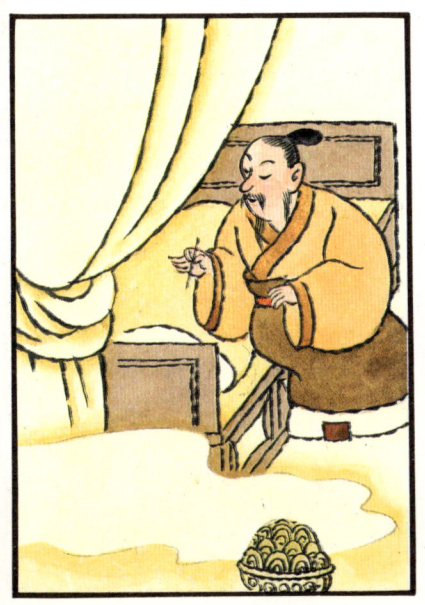
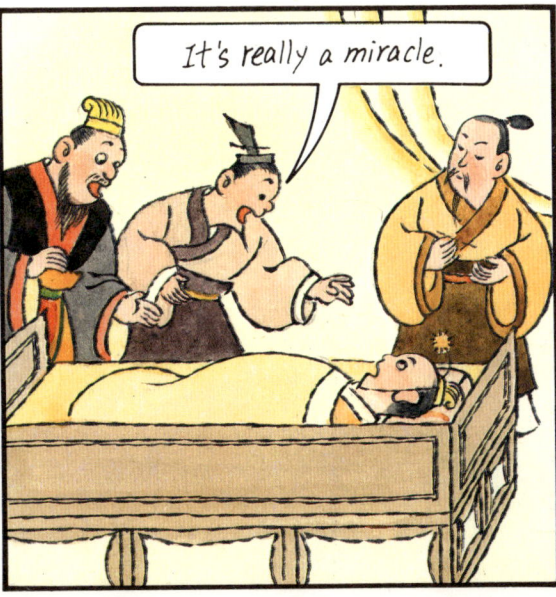
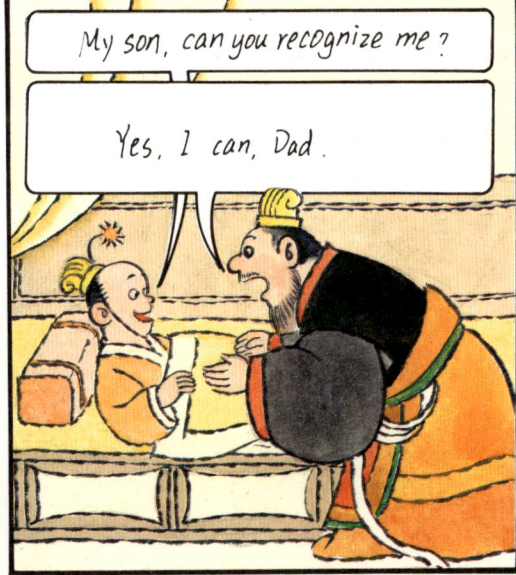

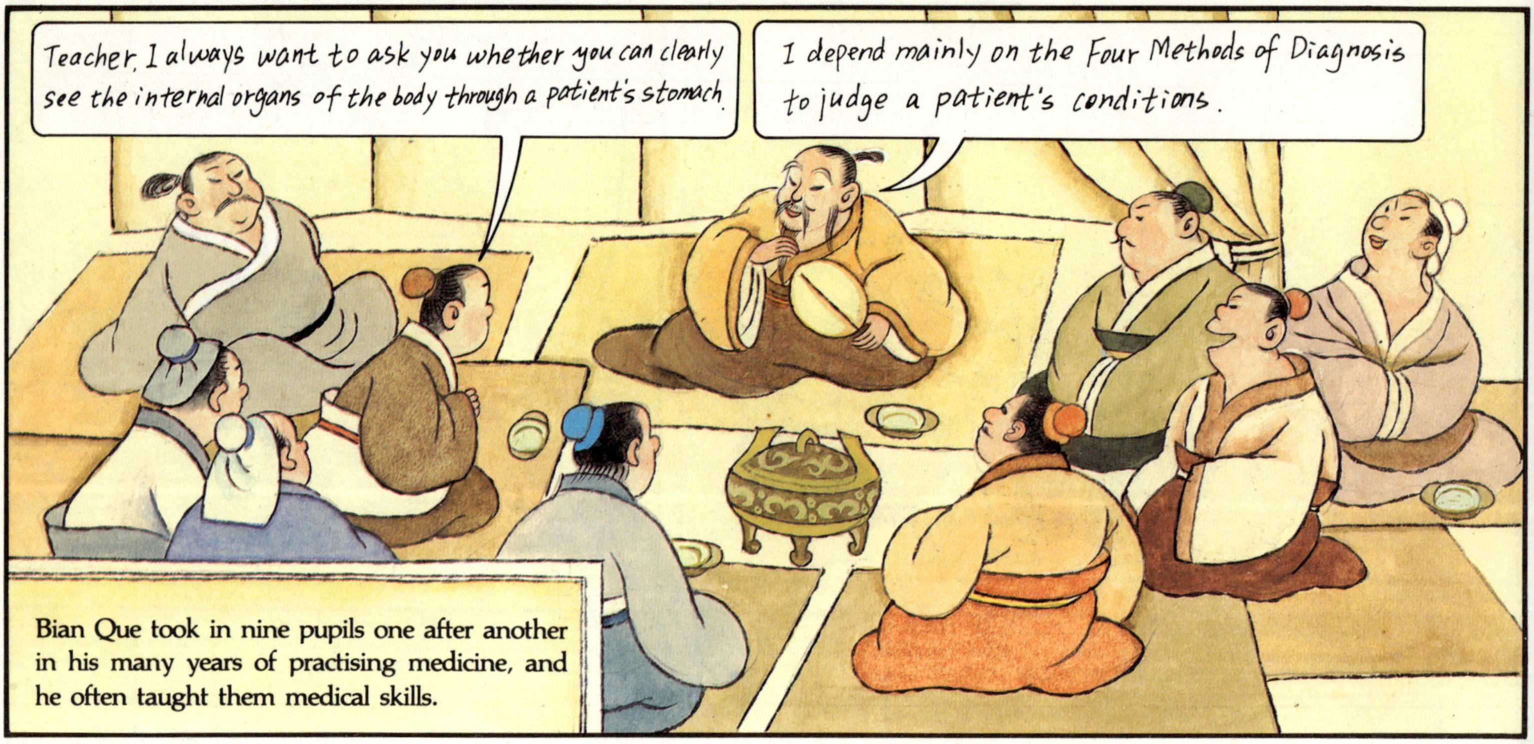

"Teacher, I always want to ask you whether you can clearly see the internal organs of the body through a patient's stomach."

"I depend mainly on the Four Methods of Diagnosis to judge a patient's conditions."

Bian Que took in nine pupils one after another in his many years of practising medicine, and he often taught them medical skills.

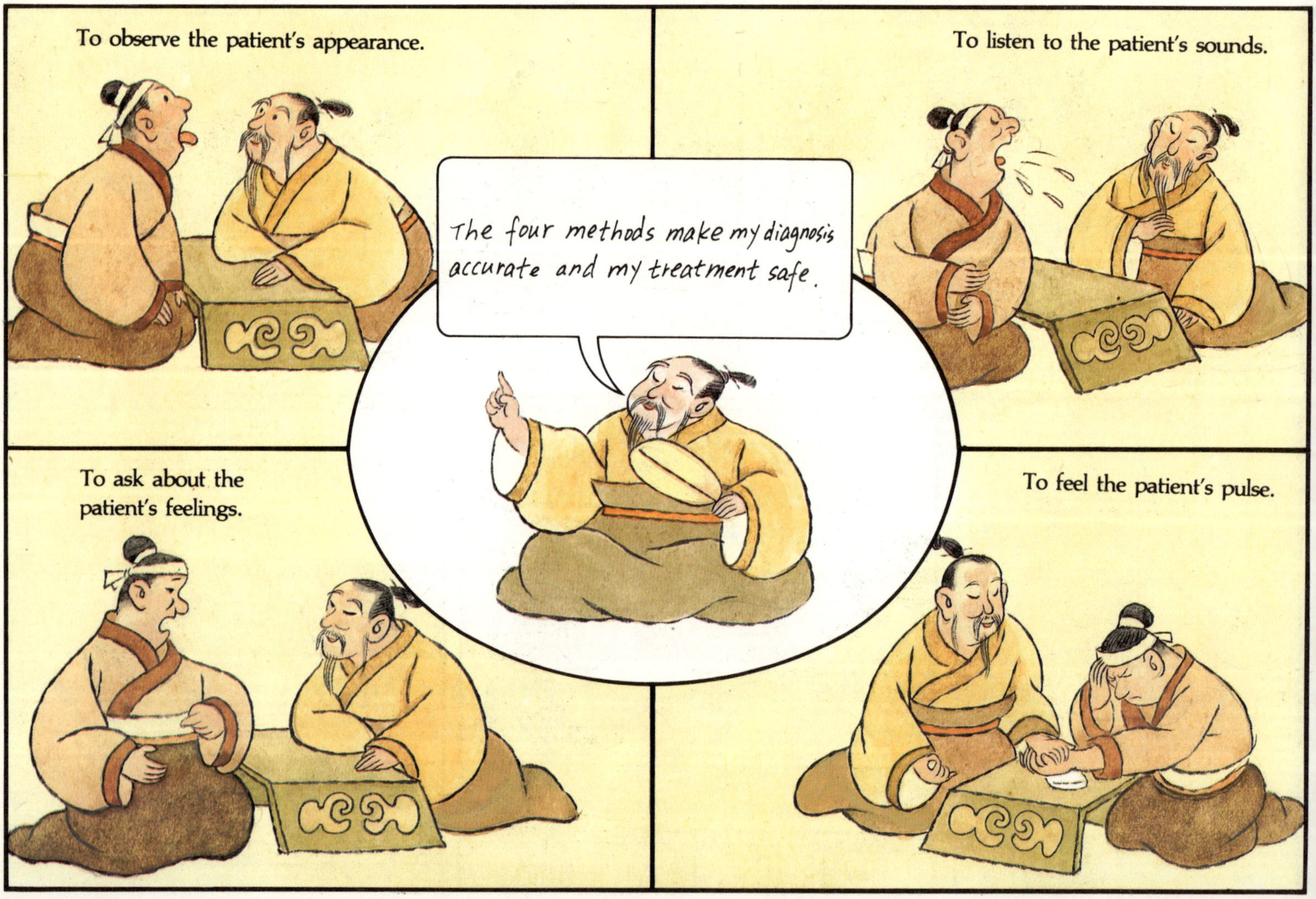

To observe the patient's appearance.

To listen to the patient's sounds.

"The four methods make my diagnosis accurate and my treatment safe."

To ask about the patient's feelings.

To feel the patient's pulse.

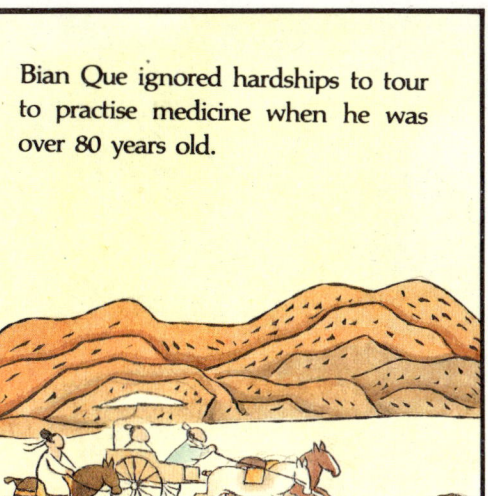
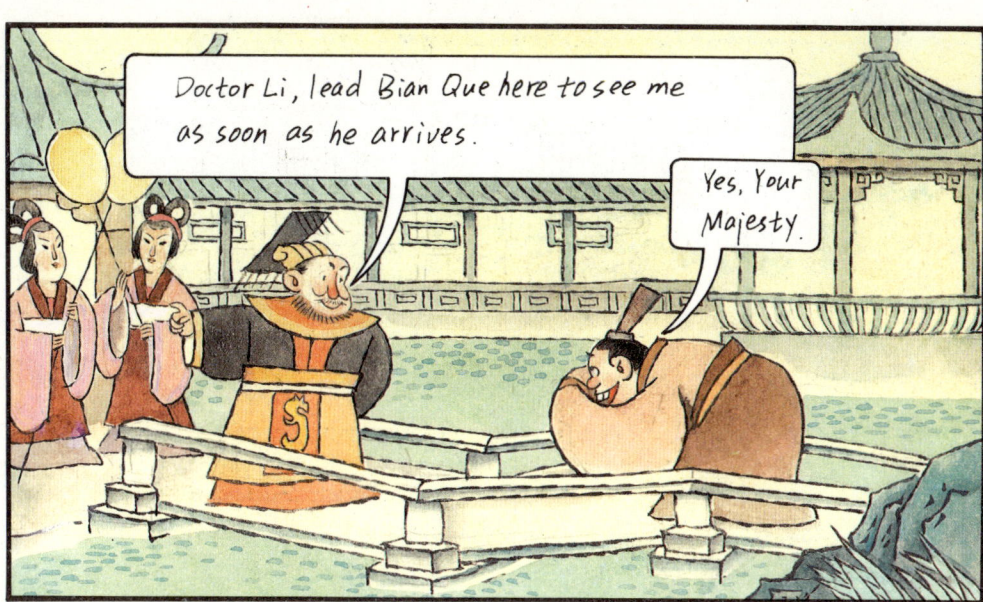
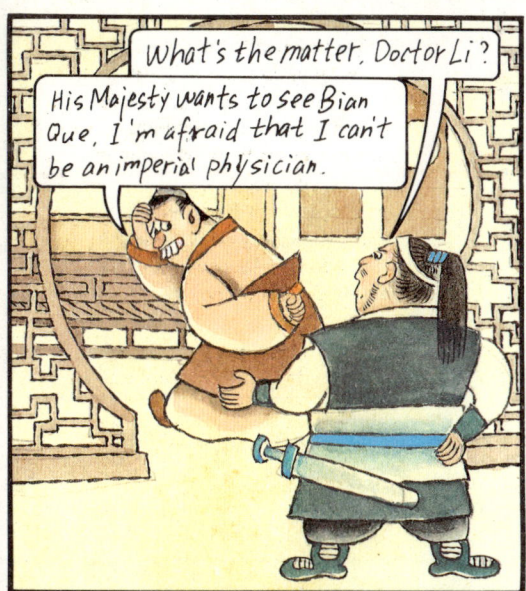
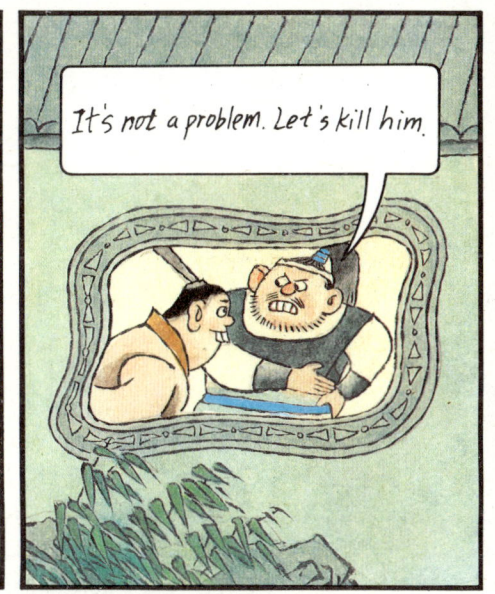
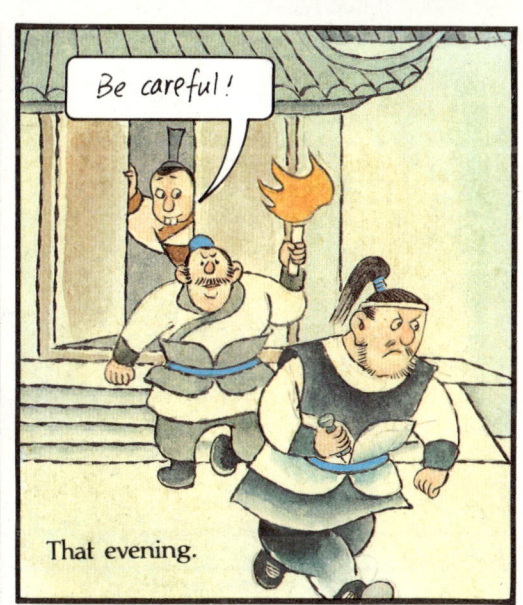
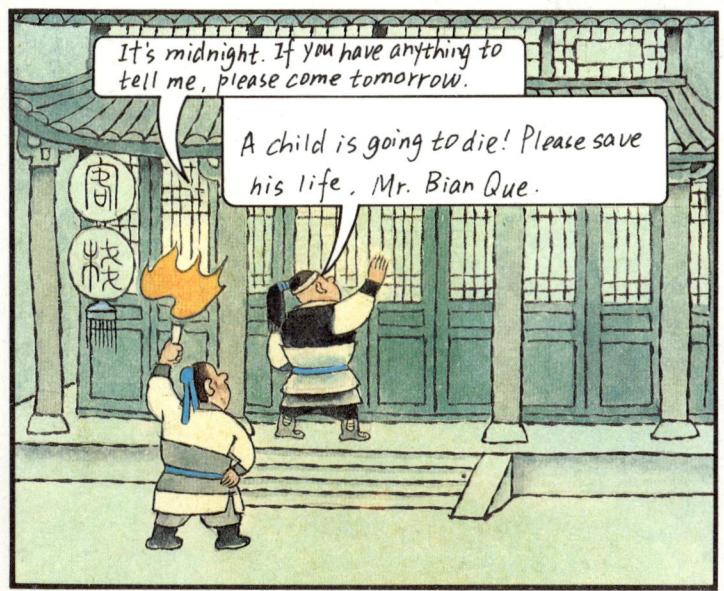
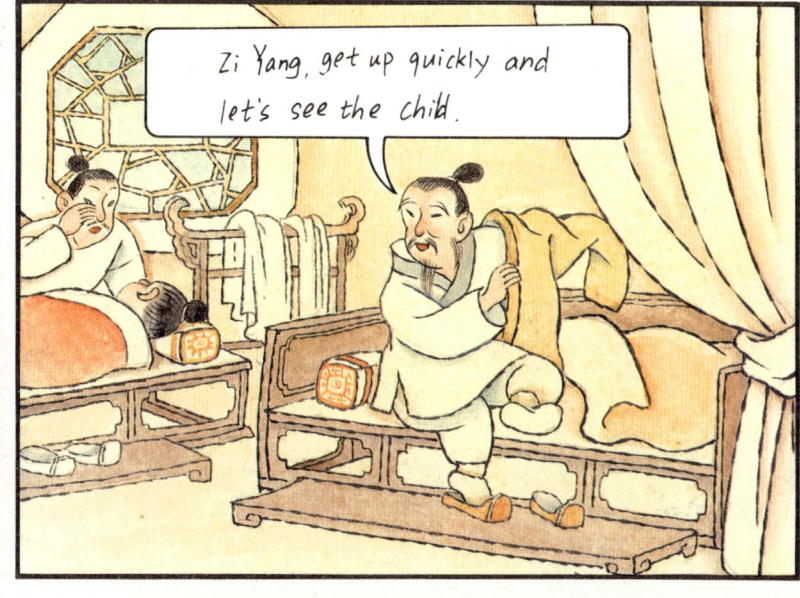

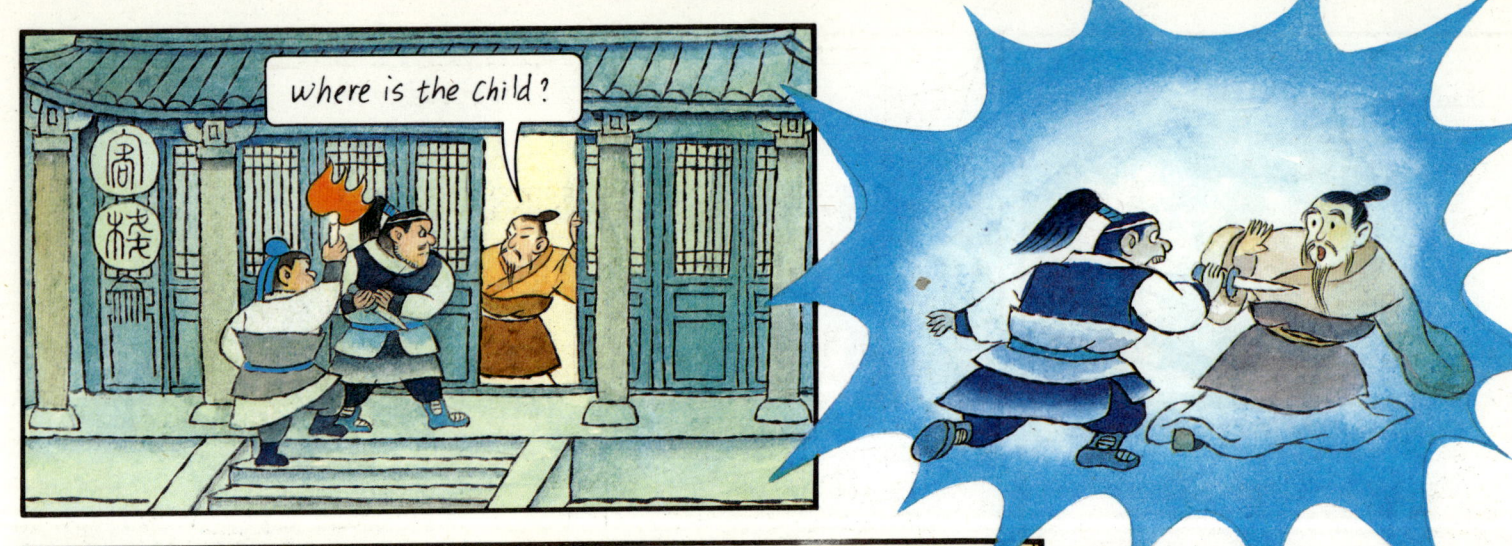

Bian Que was killed. However, he handed down his rich medical experiences to his nine pupils, who followed his principles of practising medicine.

The Principles of "Six Persons Not to Treat"
I. Not to treat those who are overbearing and self-indulgent.
II. Not to treat those who care for money more than their health.
III. Not to treat those who cannot take care of themselves.
IV. Not to treat those who have both *yin* and *yang qi* (vital energy).
V. Not to treat those who are thin and weak, and cannot take medicine.
VI. Not to treat those who believe in sorcery but not in medicine.

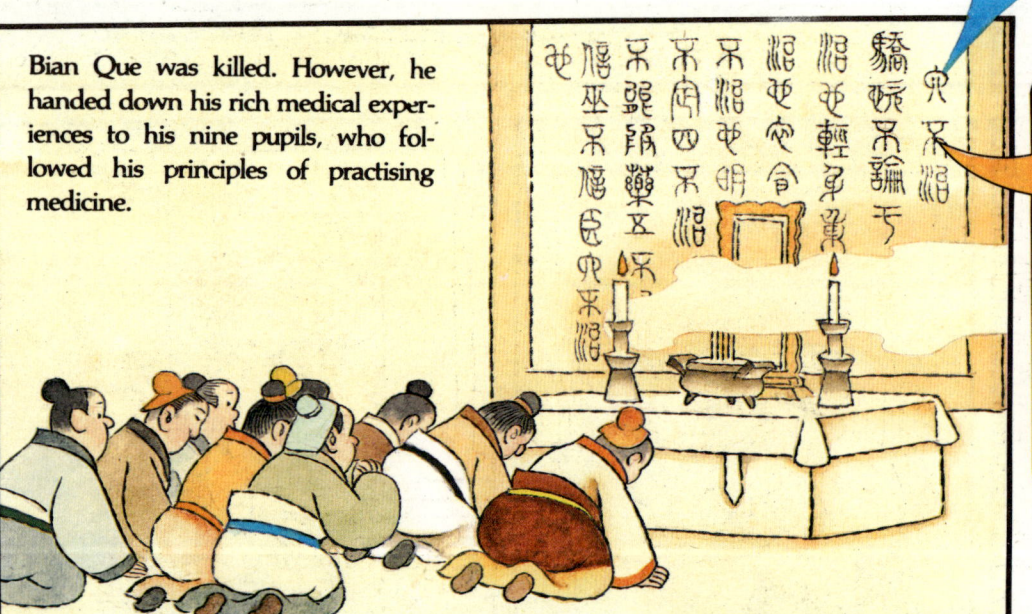

By the Han Dynasty, Bian Que's medical theories and experiences were summed up into a classical medical work entitled *Huangdi's Classic on 81 Medical Problems*, which exerted a great influence on the development of medical sciences of later generations.

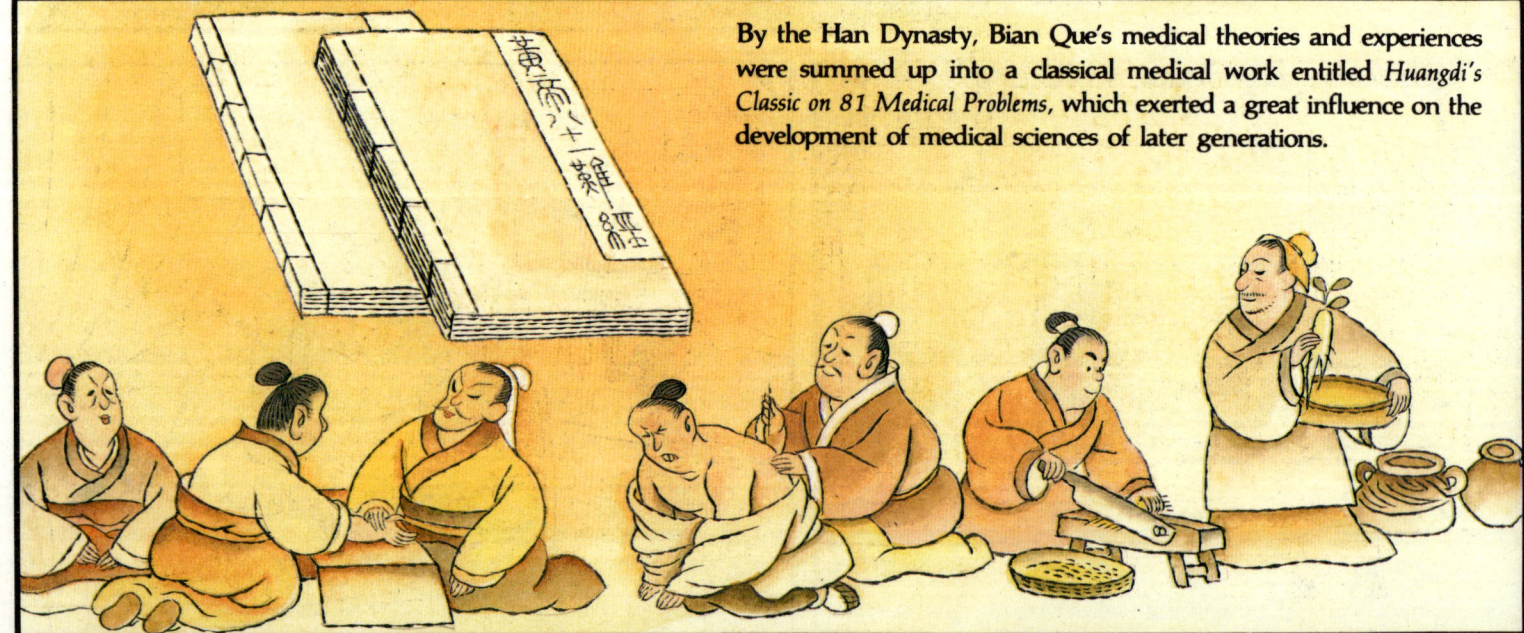

HUA TUO

A distinguished doctor of ancient China, Hua Tuo (145-208) made remarkable achievements in the diagnosis of diseases and health care, as well as being the first in the world to do surgical operations of the abdominal cavity using anaesthesia.

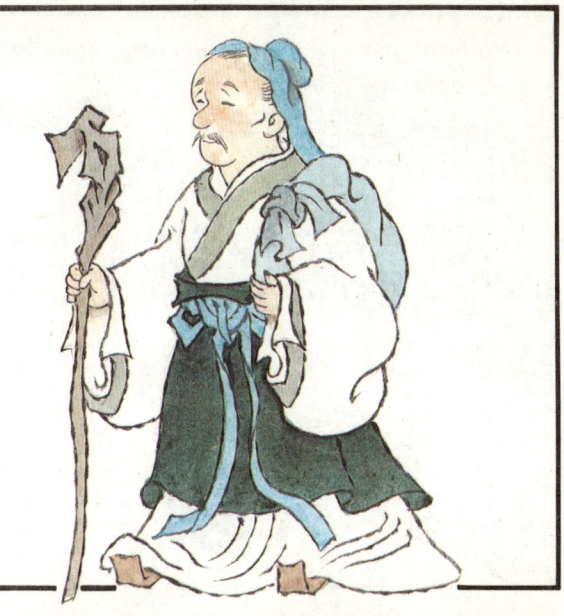

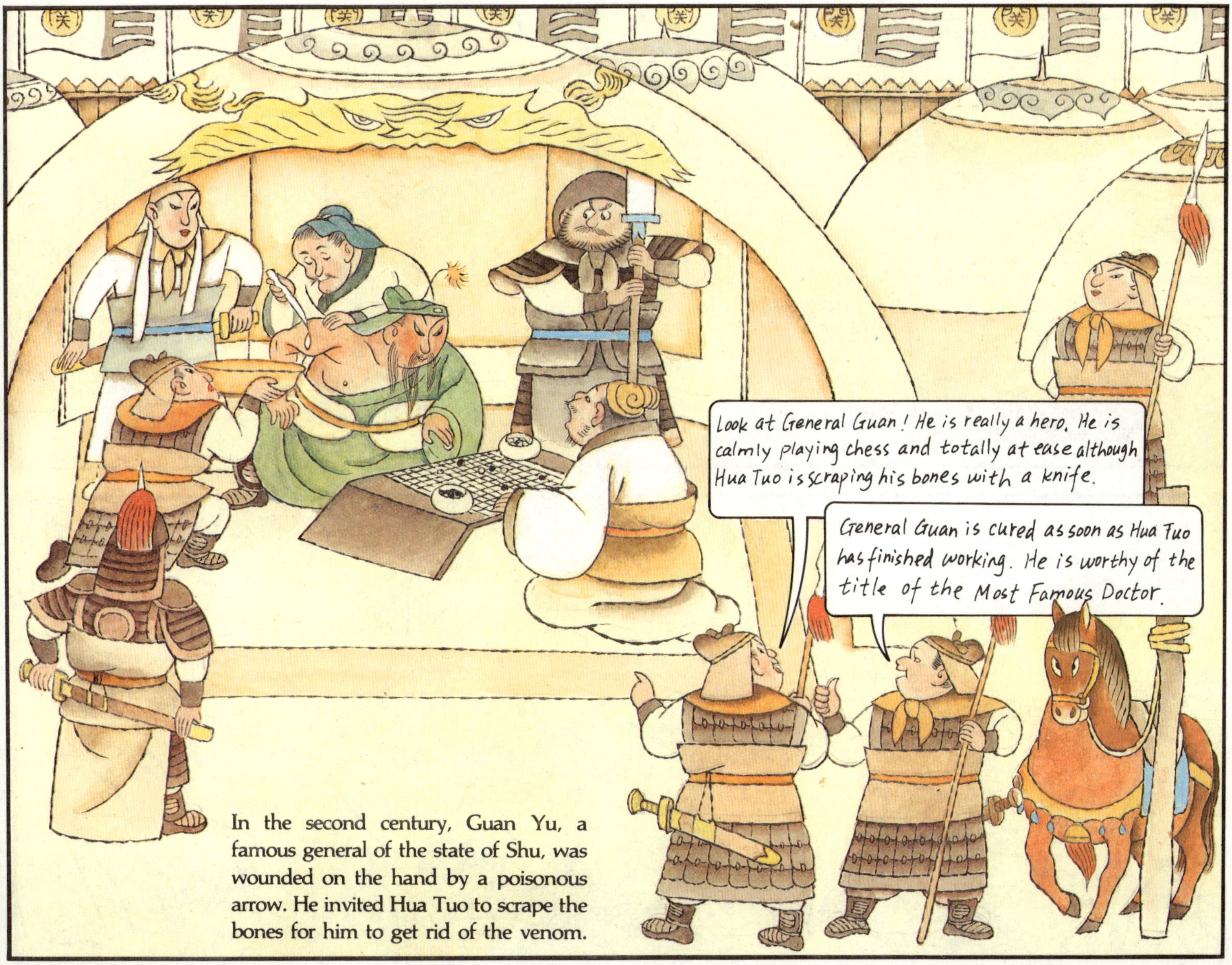

In the second century, Guan Yu, a famous general of the state of Shu, was wounded on the hand by a poisonous arrow. He invited Hua Tuo to scrape the bones for him to get rid of the venom.

Look at General Guan! He is really a hero. He is calmly playing chess and totally at ease although Hua Tuo is scraping his bones with a knife.

General Guan is cured as soon as Hua Tuo has finished working. He is worthy of the title of the Most Famous Doctor.

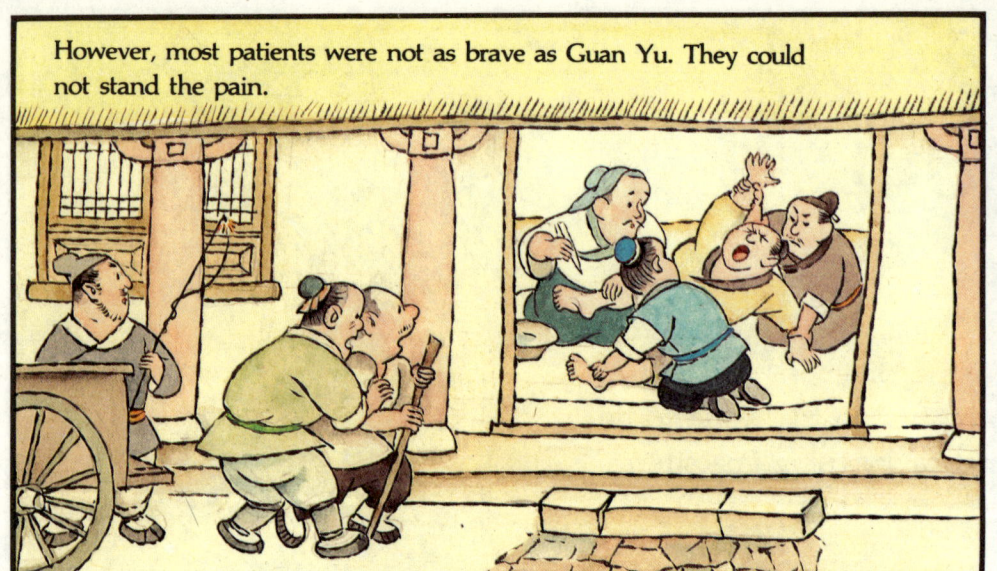
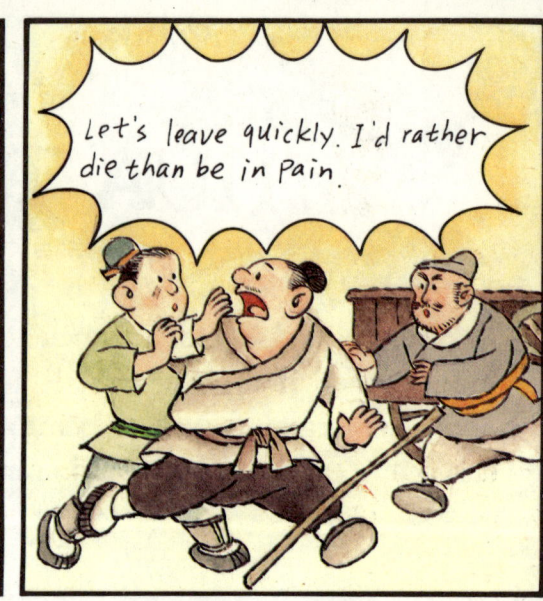
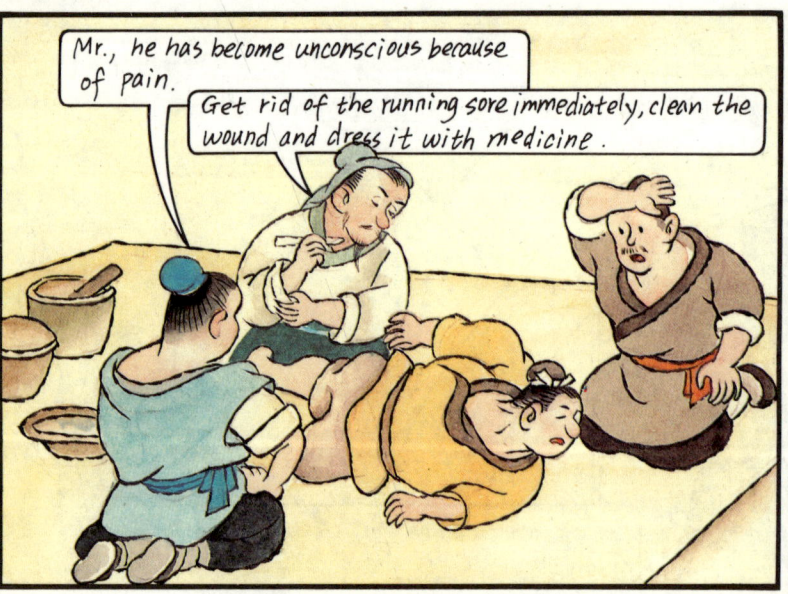
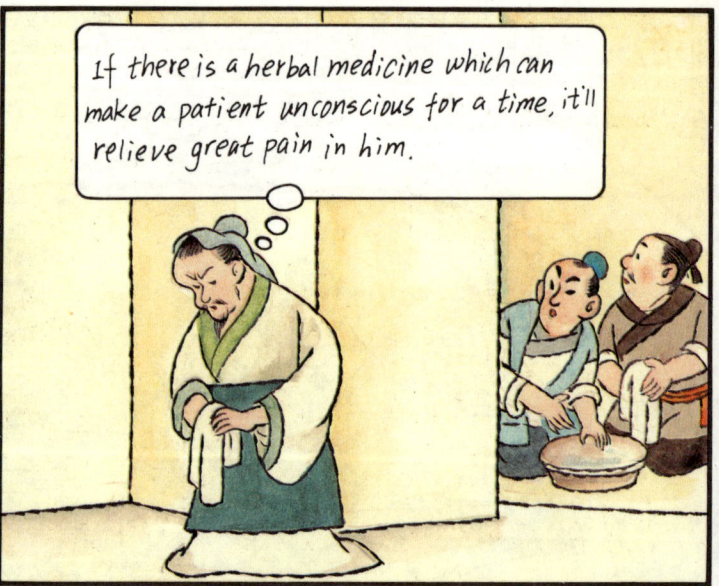
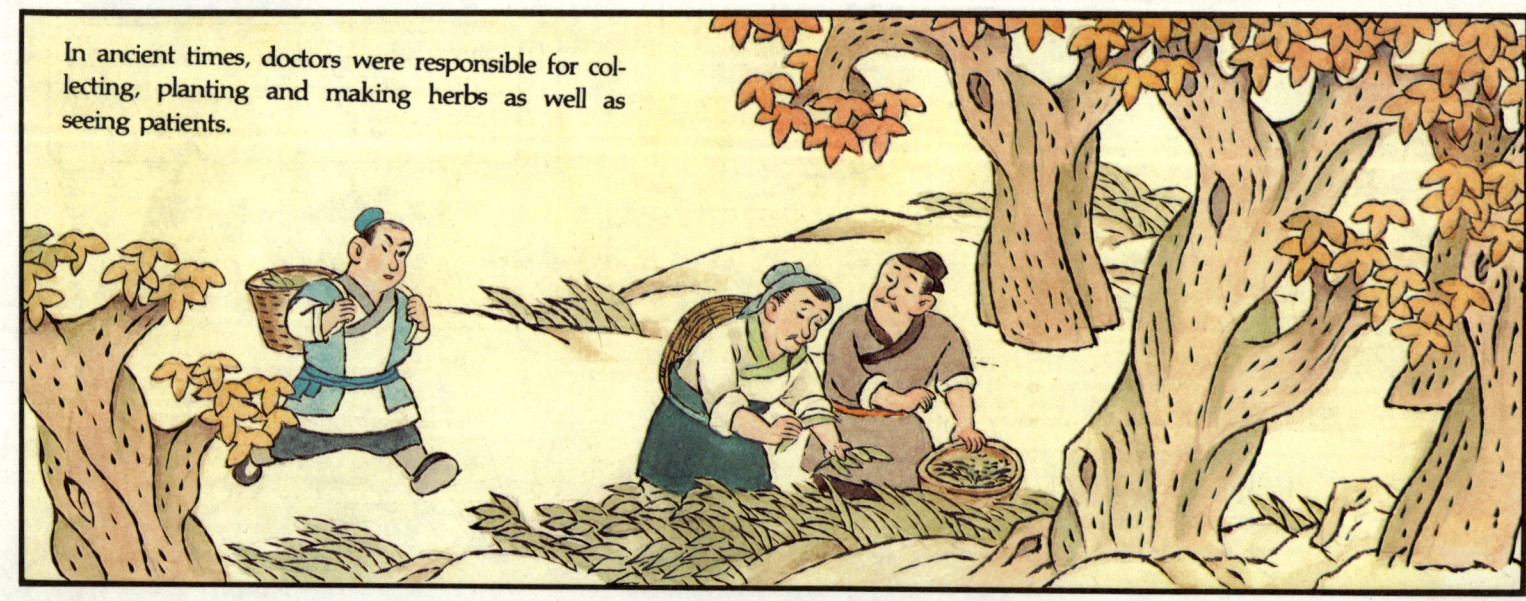

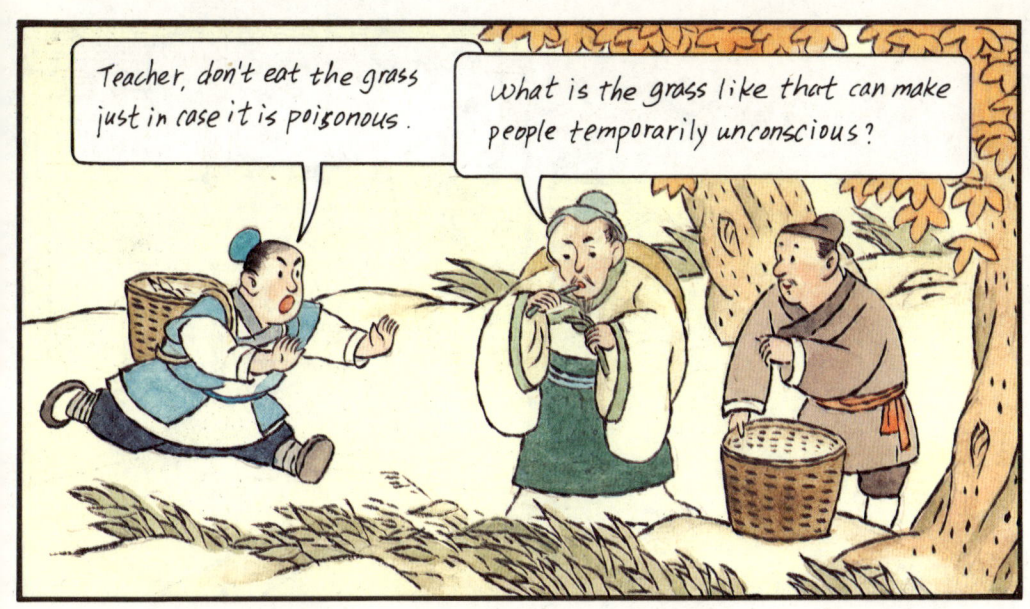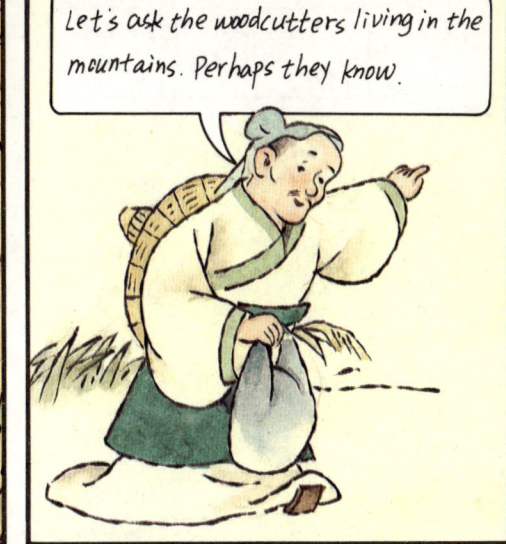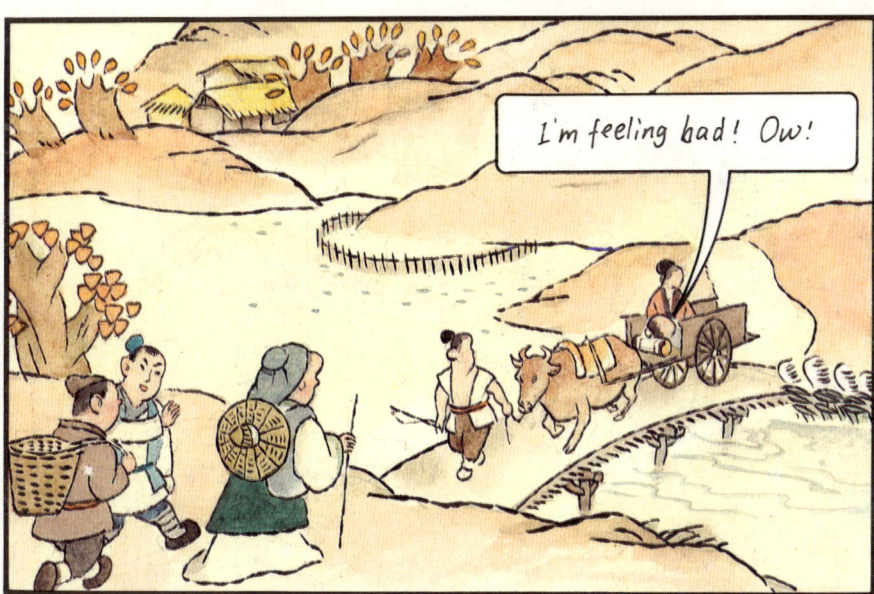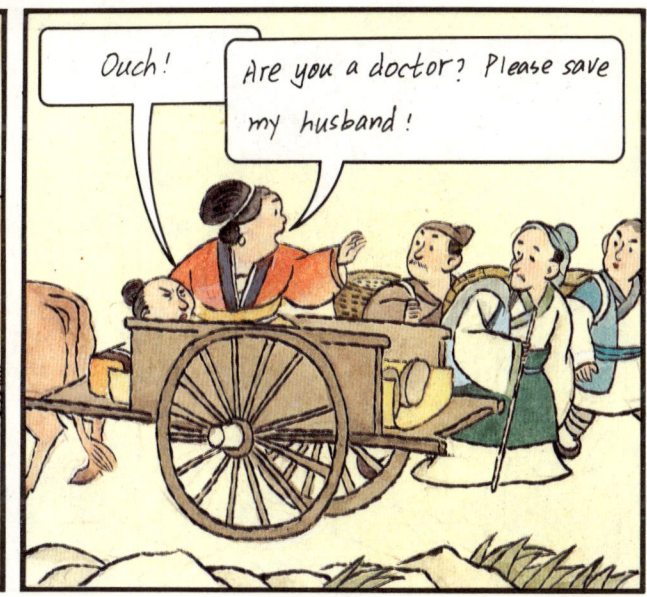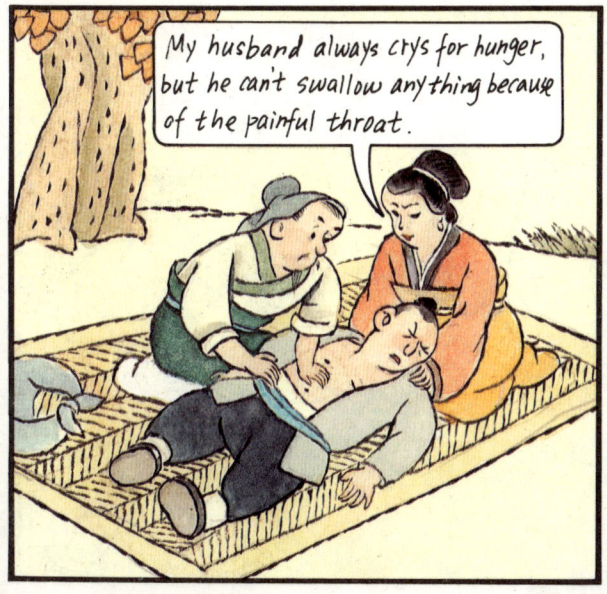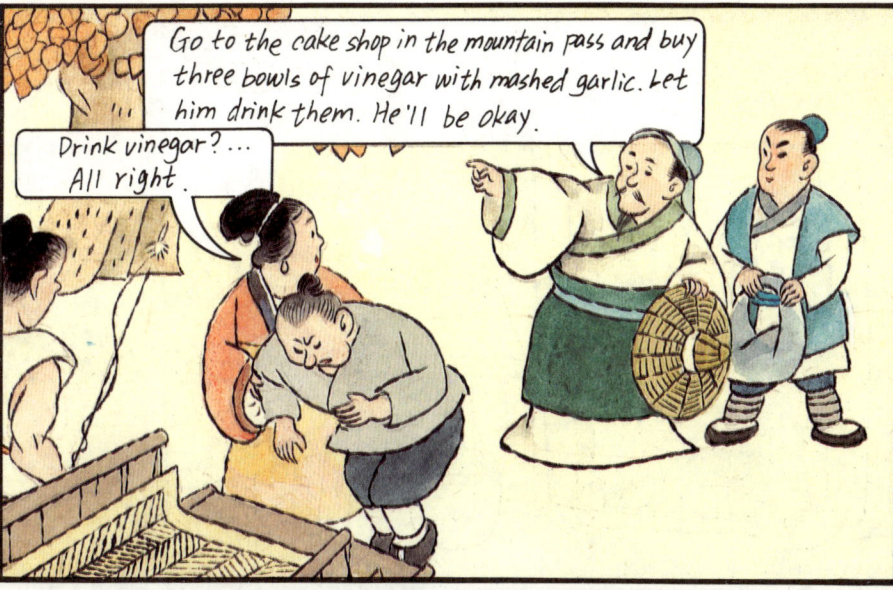

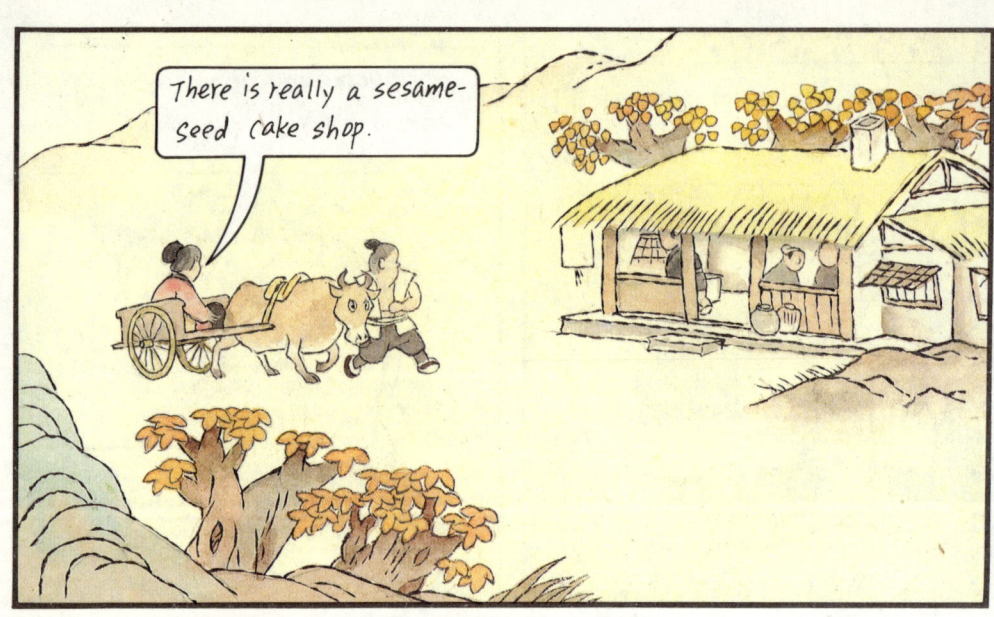
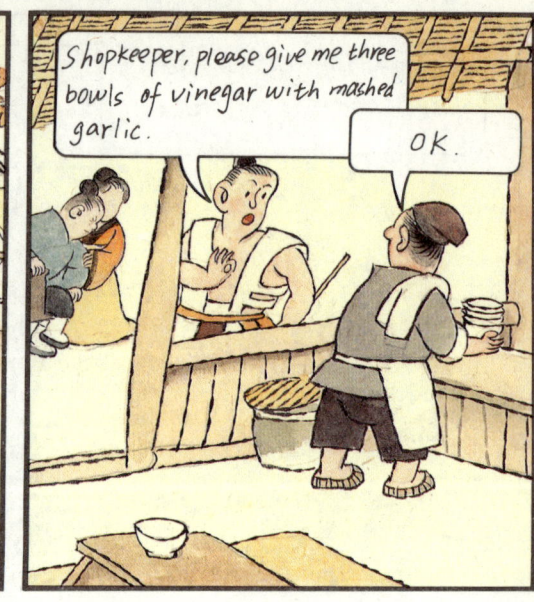
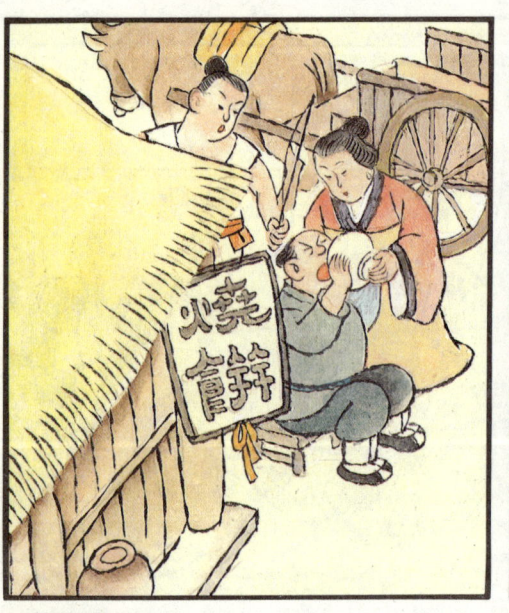
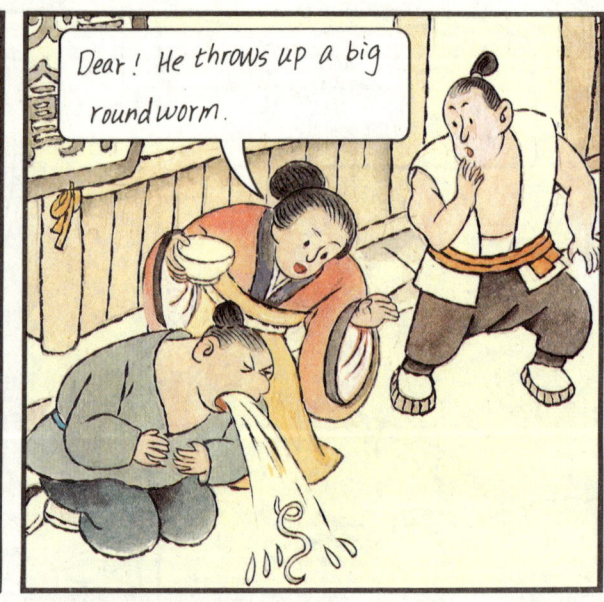
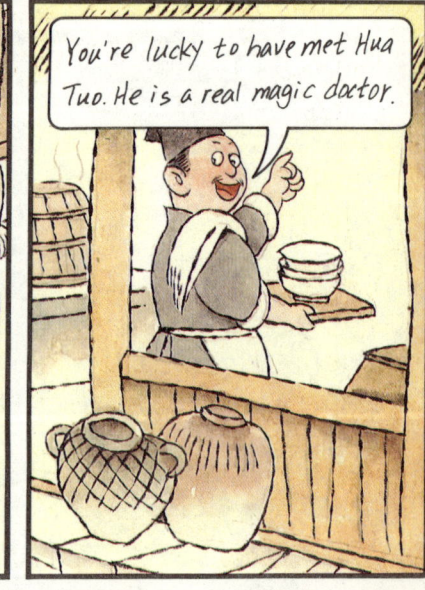
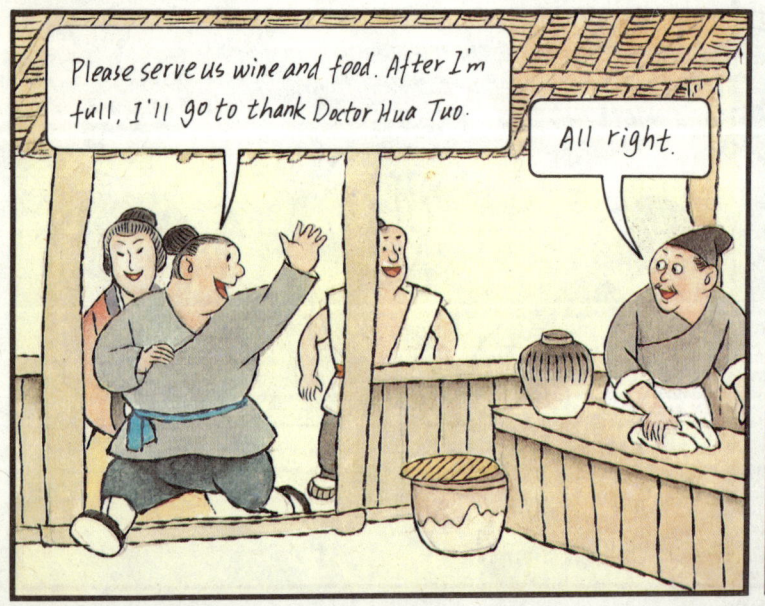
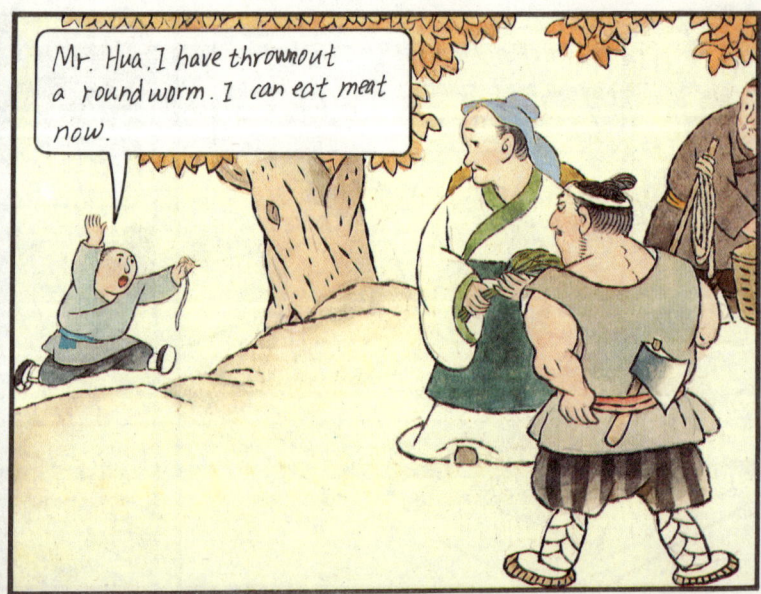

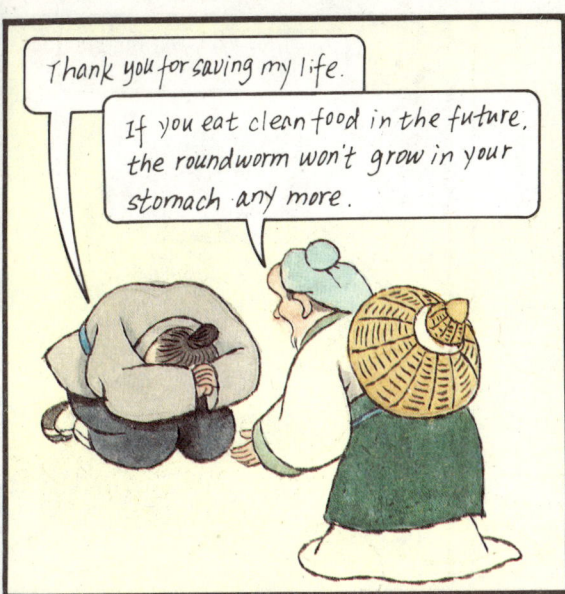
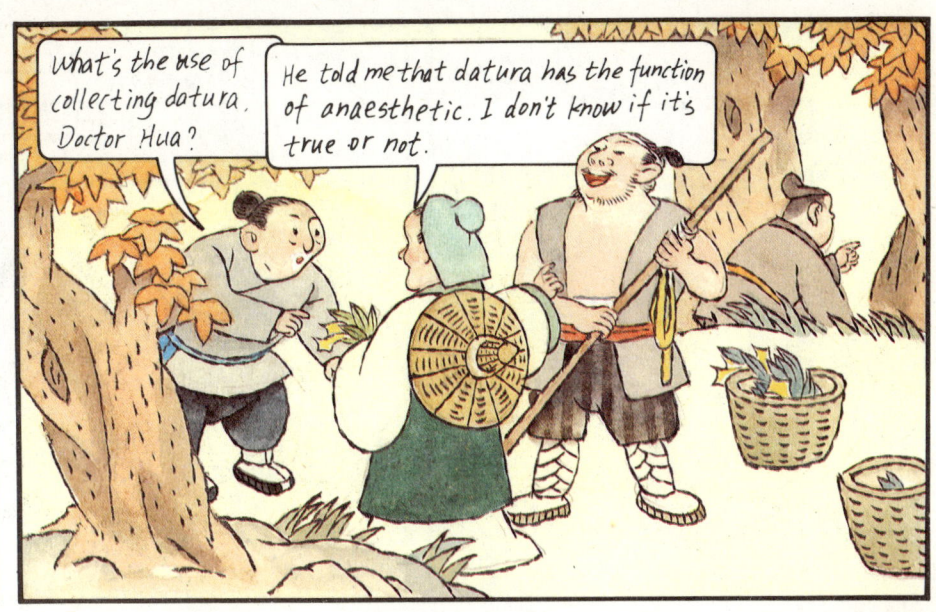
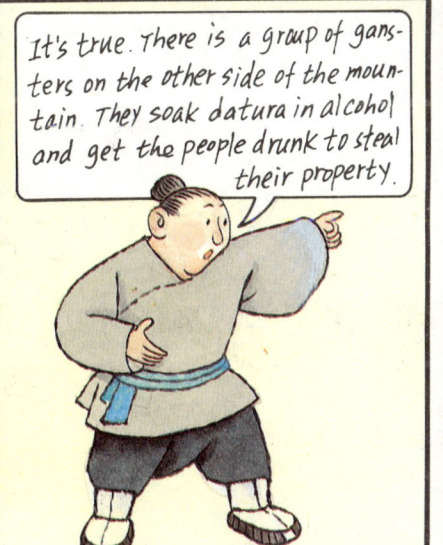
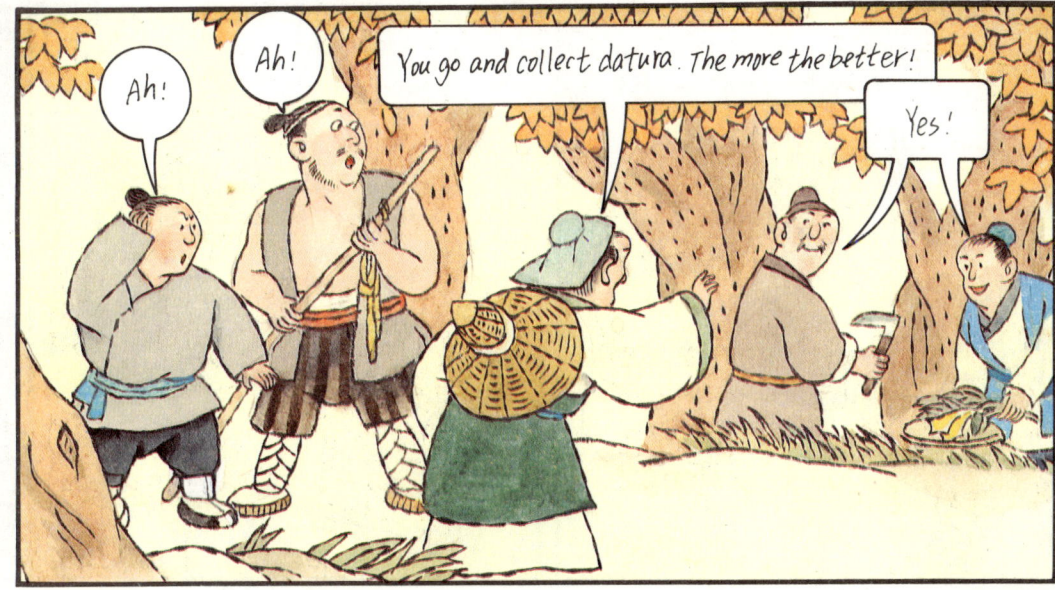
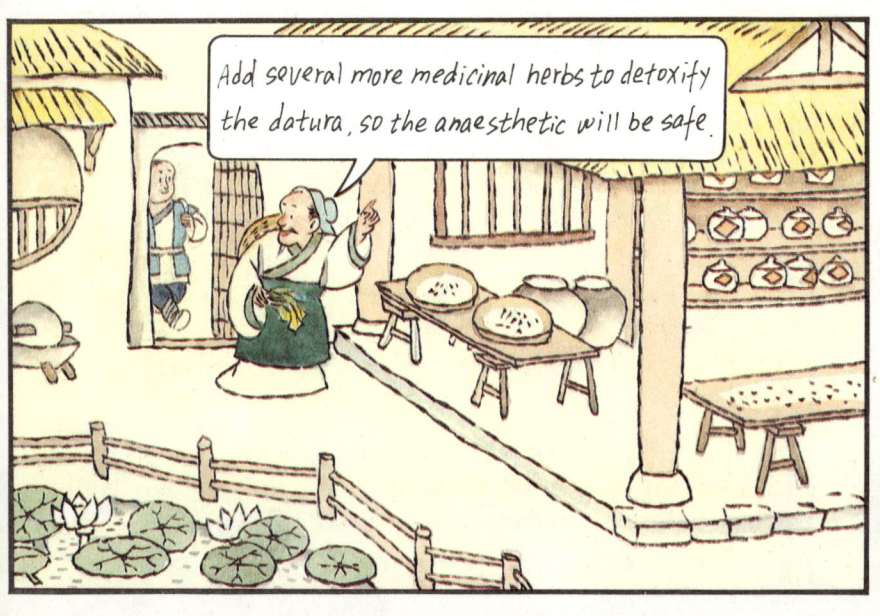
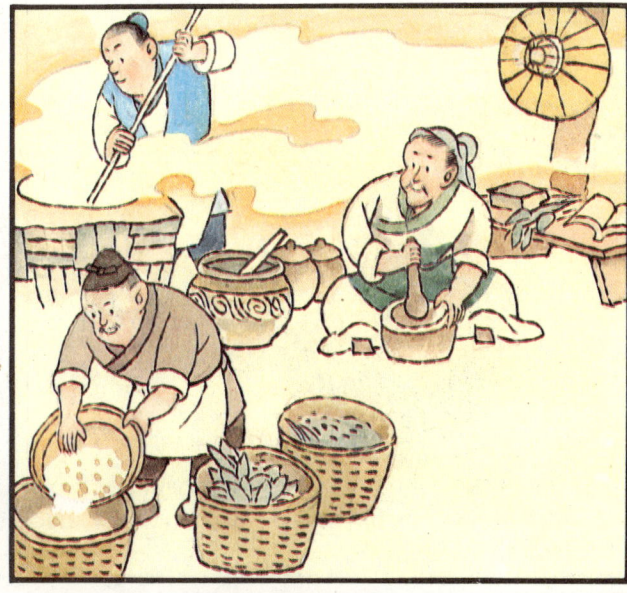

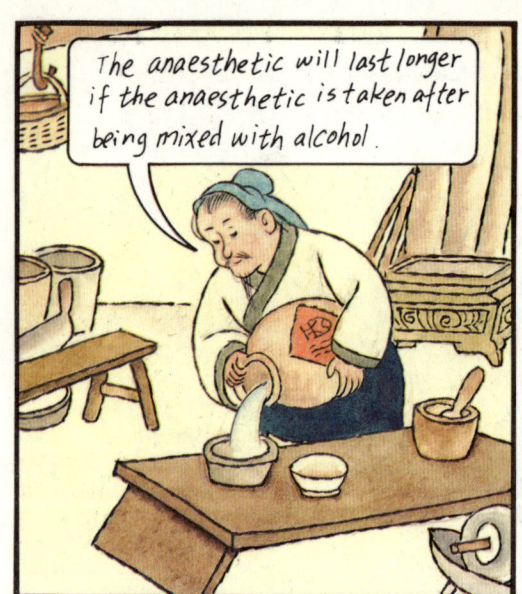
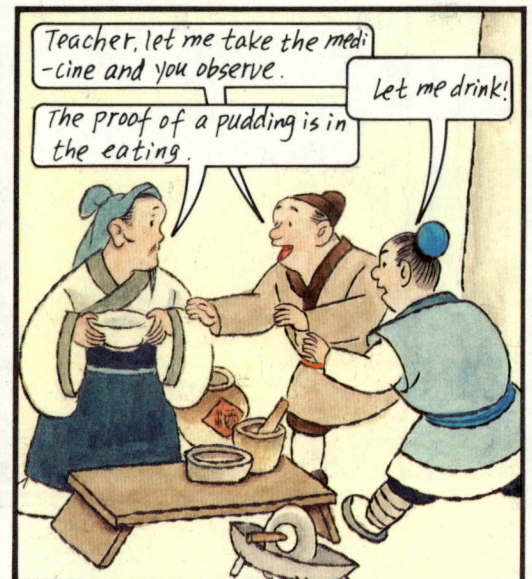
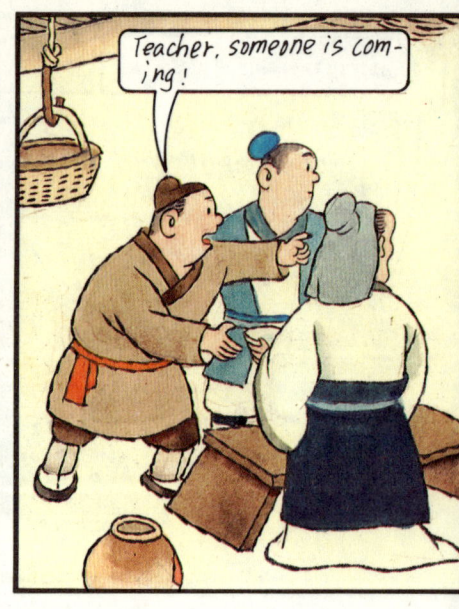
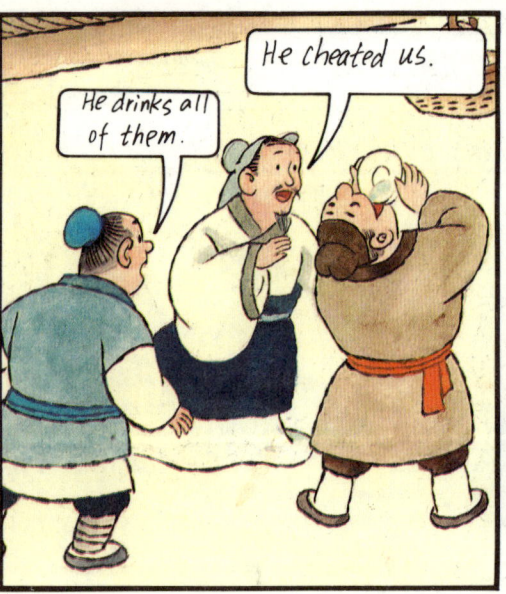
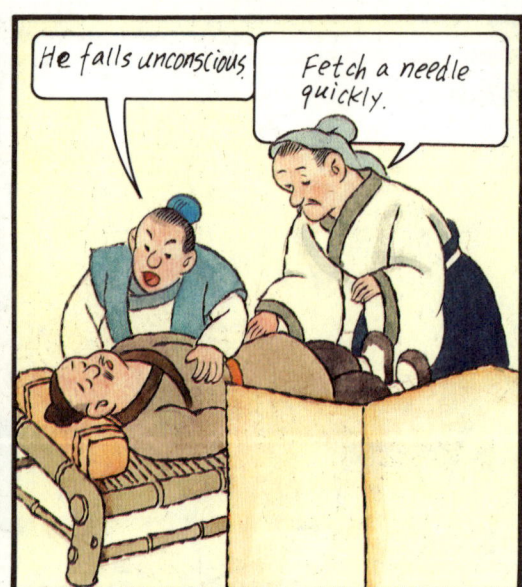
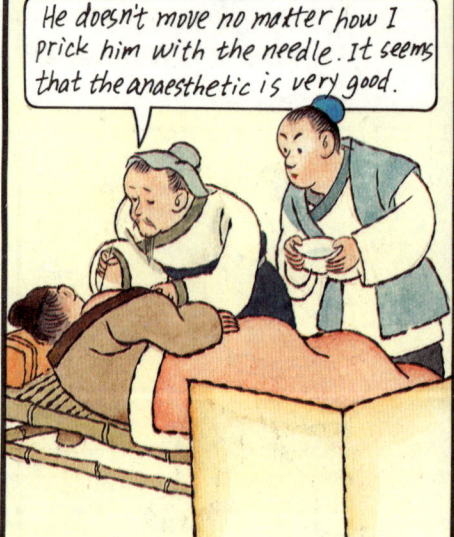

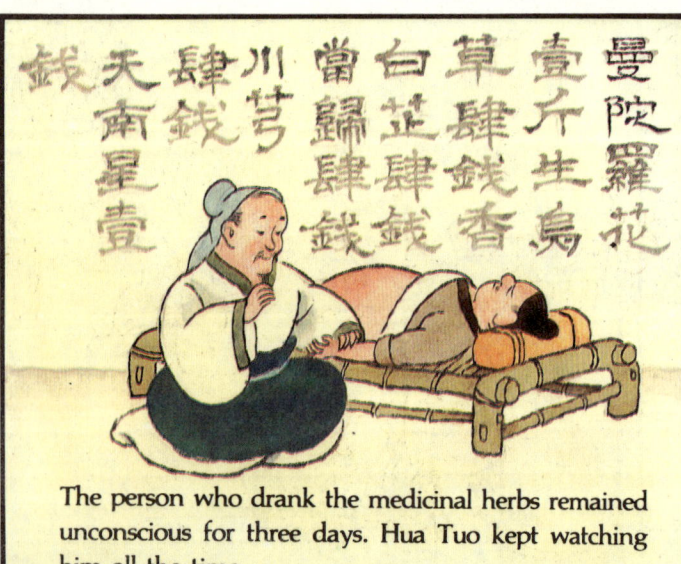

The person who drank the medicinal herbs remained unconscious for three days. Hua Tuo kept watching him all the time.

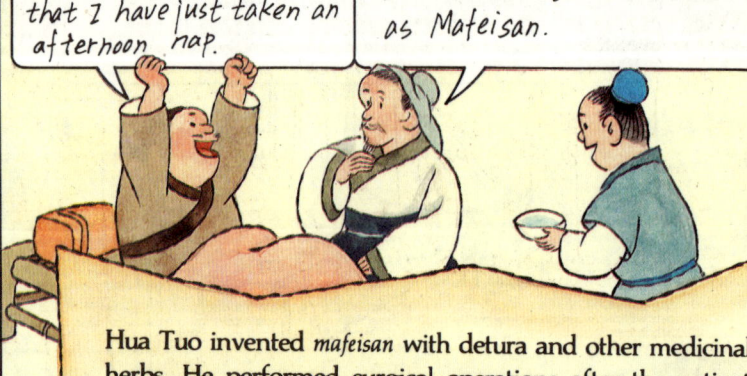

Hua Tuo invented *mafeisan* with detura and other medicinal herbs. He performed surgical operations after the patient was anaesthetized. This occurred 1,700 years ago, but the Western anaesthesia was applied to the patient only less than two hundred years ago.

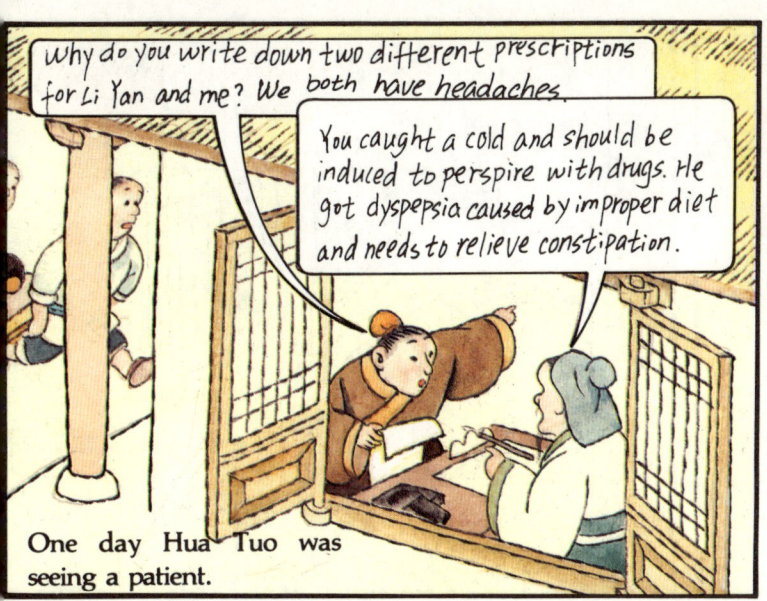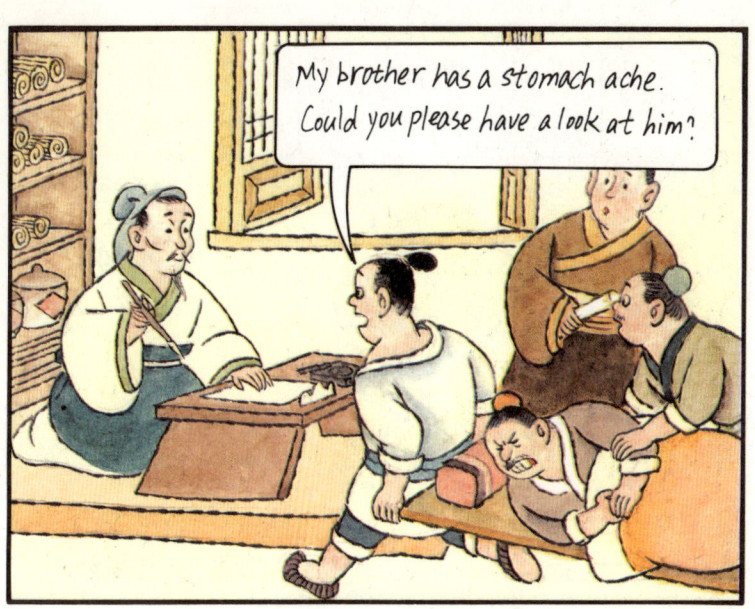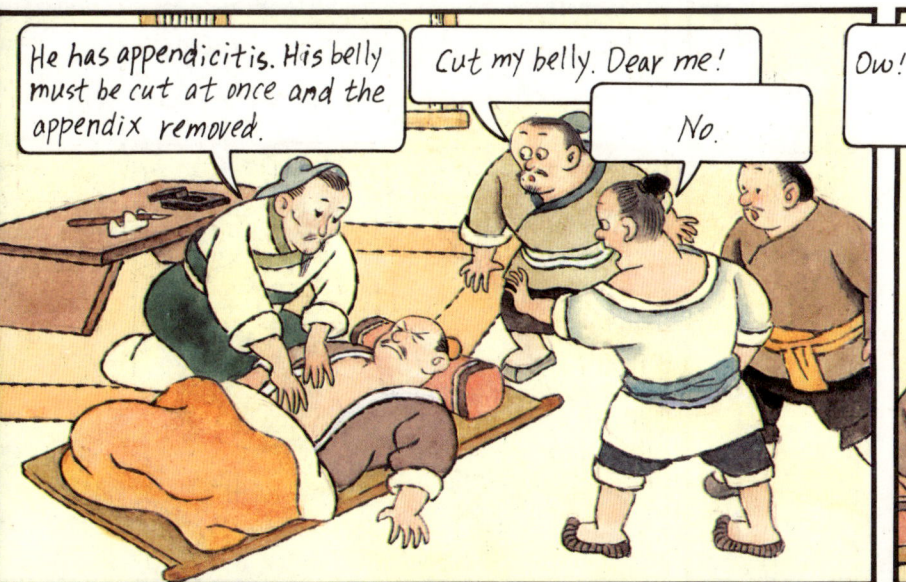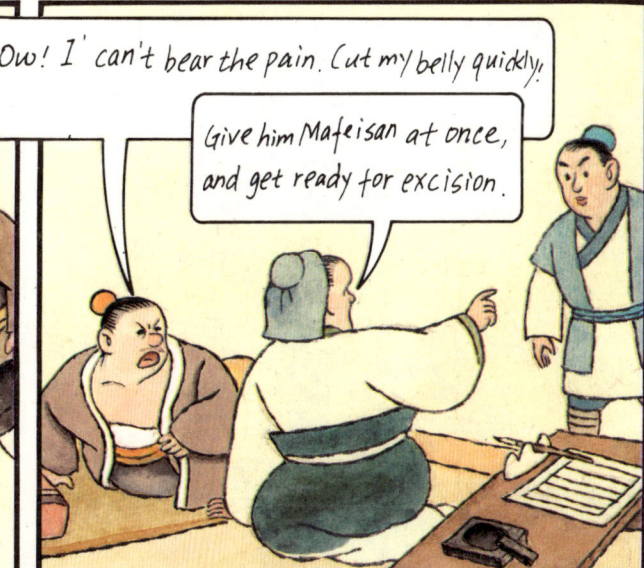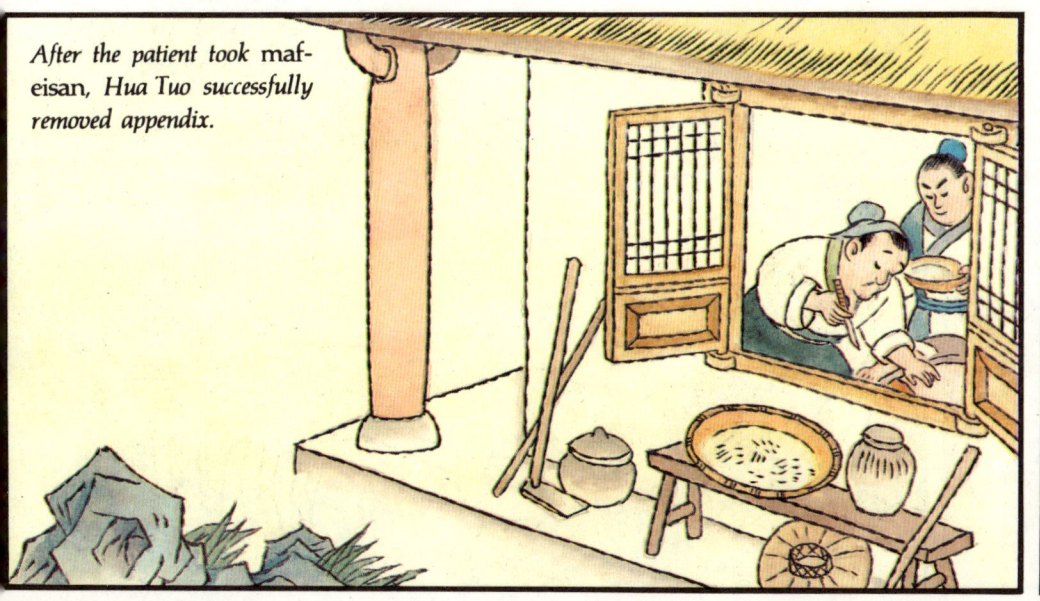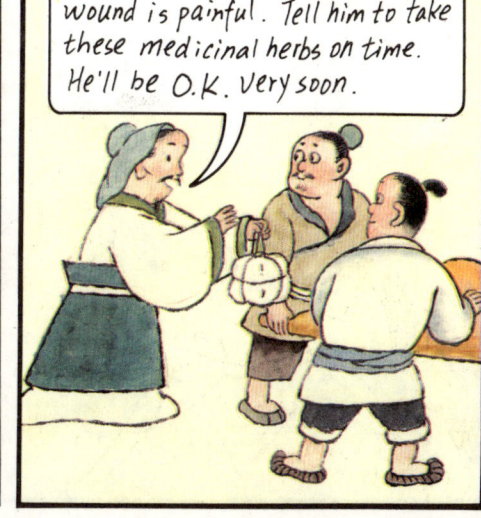

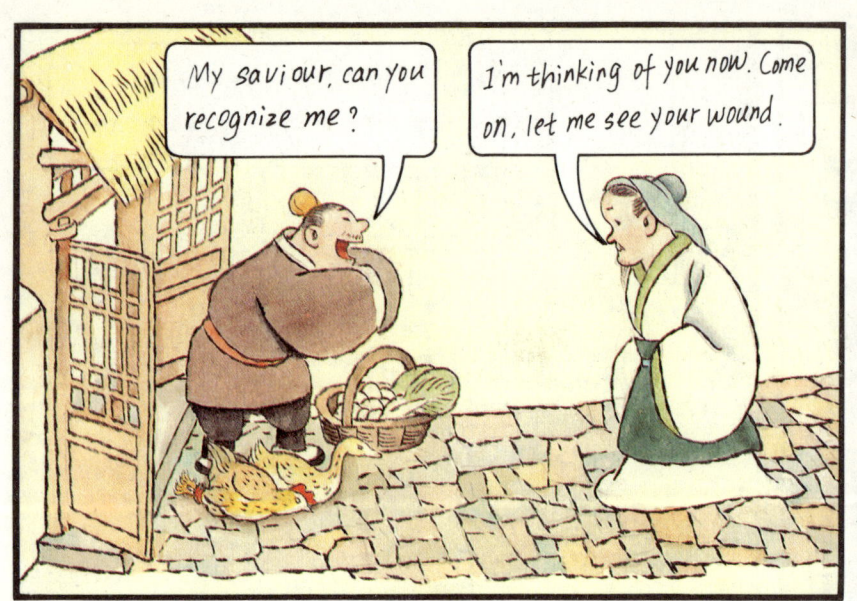
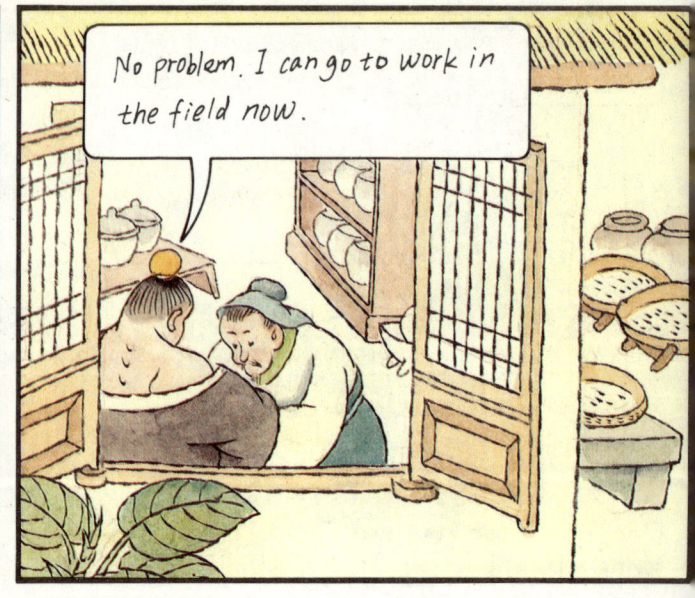
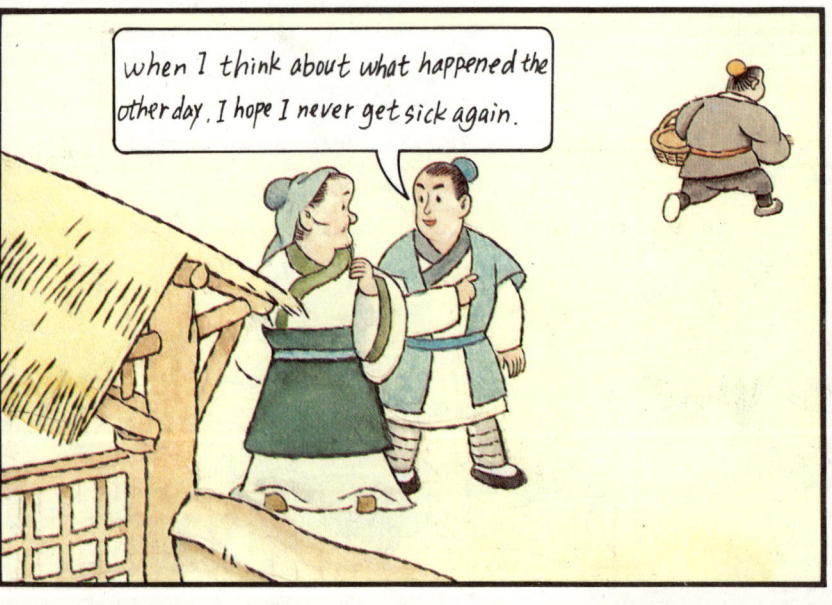
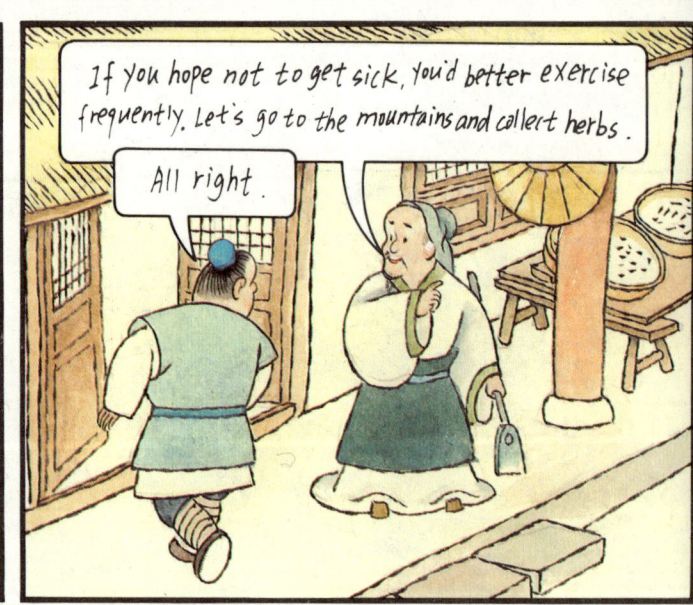
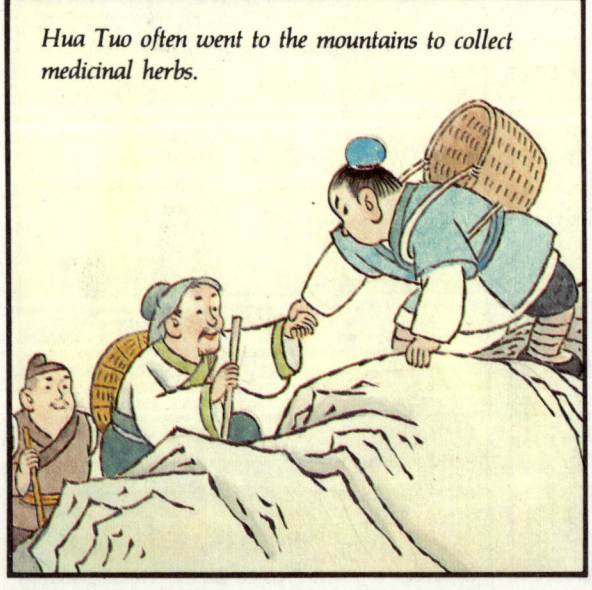

Hua Tuo often went to the mountains to collect medicinal herbs.

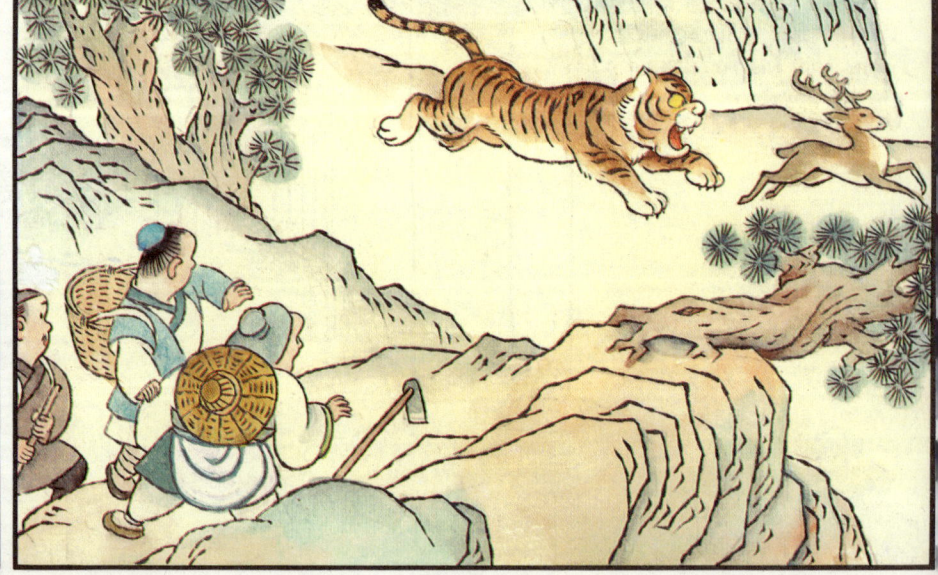

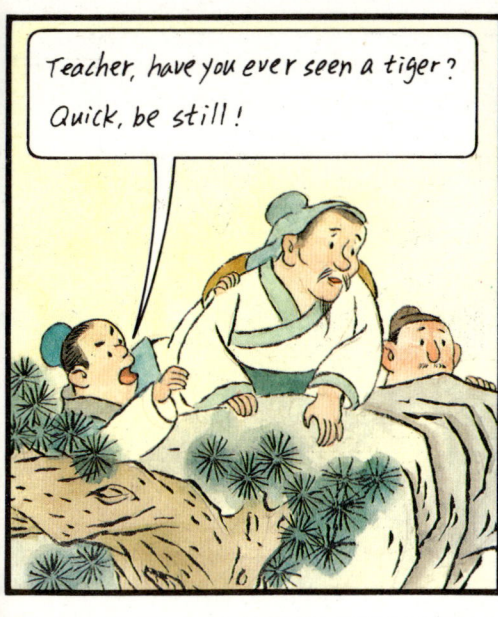
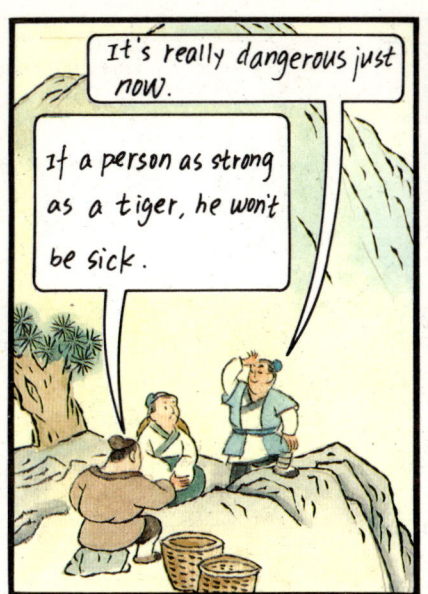
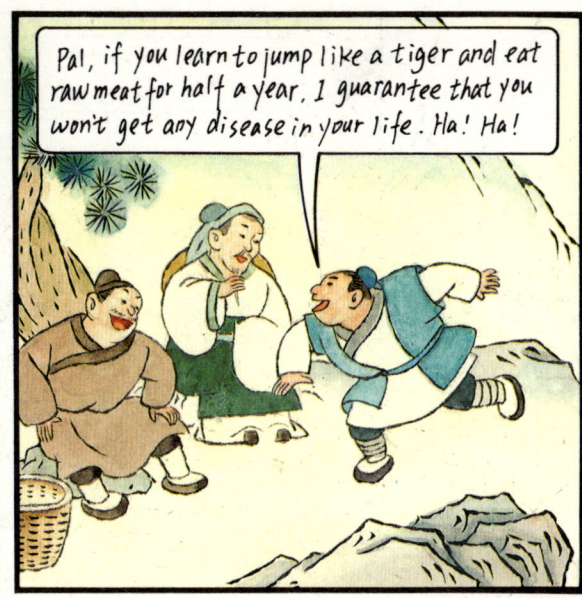
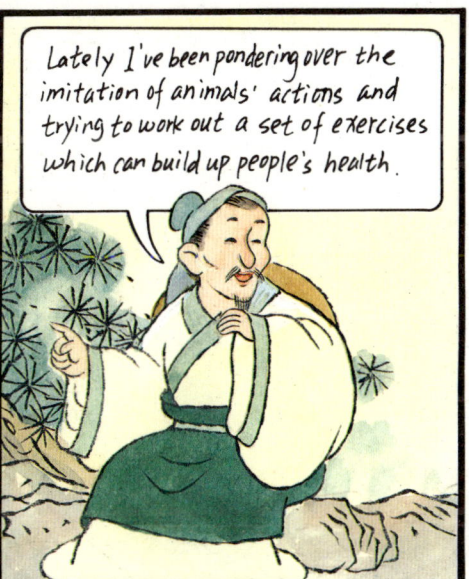
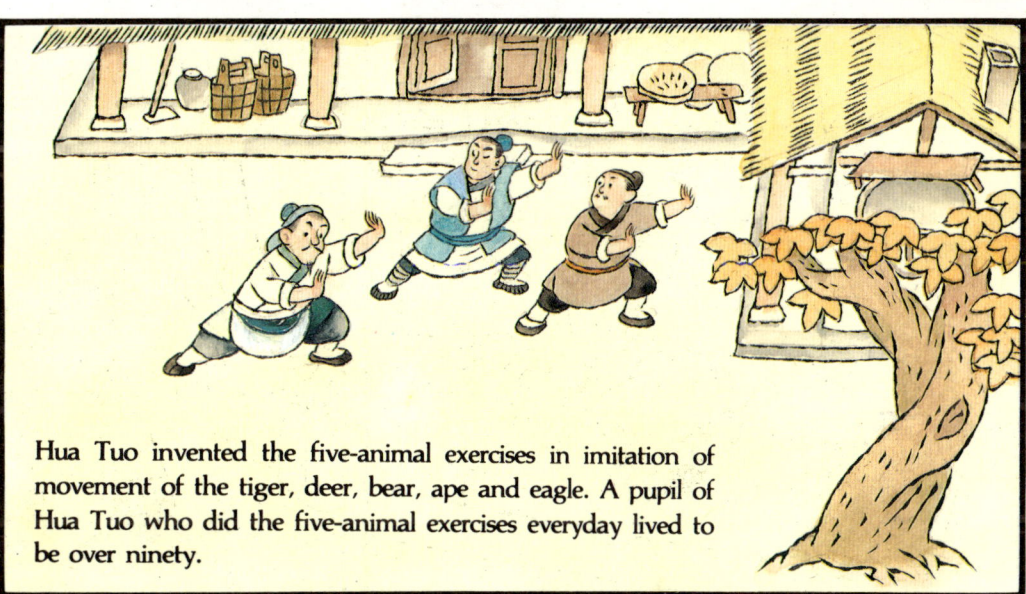

Hua Tuo invented the five-animal exercises in imitation of movement of the tiger, deer, bear, ape and eagle. A pupil of Hua Tuo who did the five-animal exercises everyday lived to be over ninety.

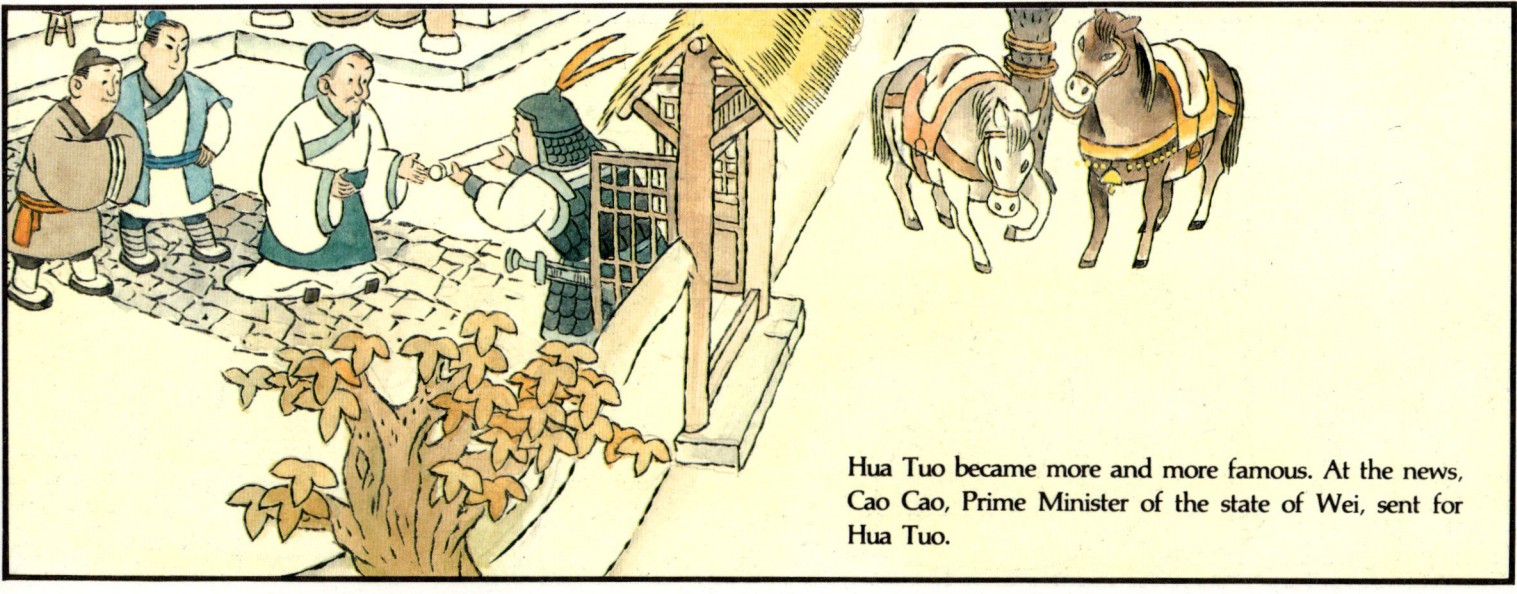

Hua Tuo became more and more famous. At the news, Cao Cao, Prime Minister of the state of Wei, sent for Hua Tuo.

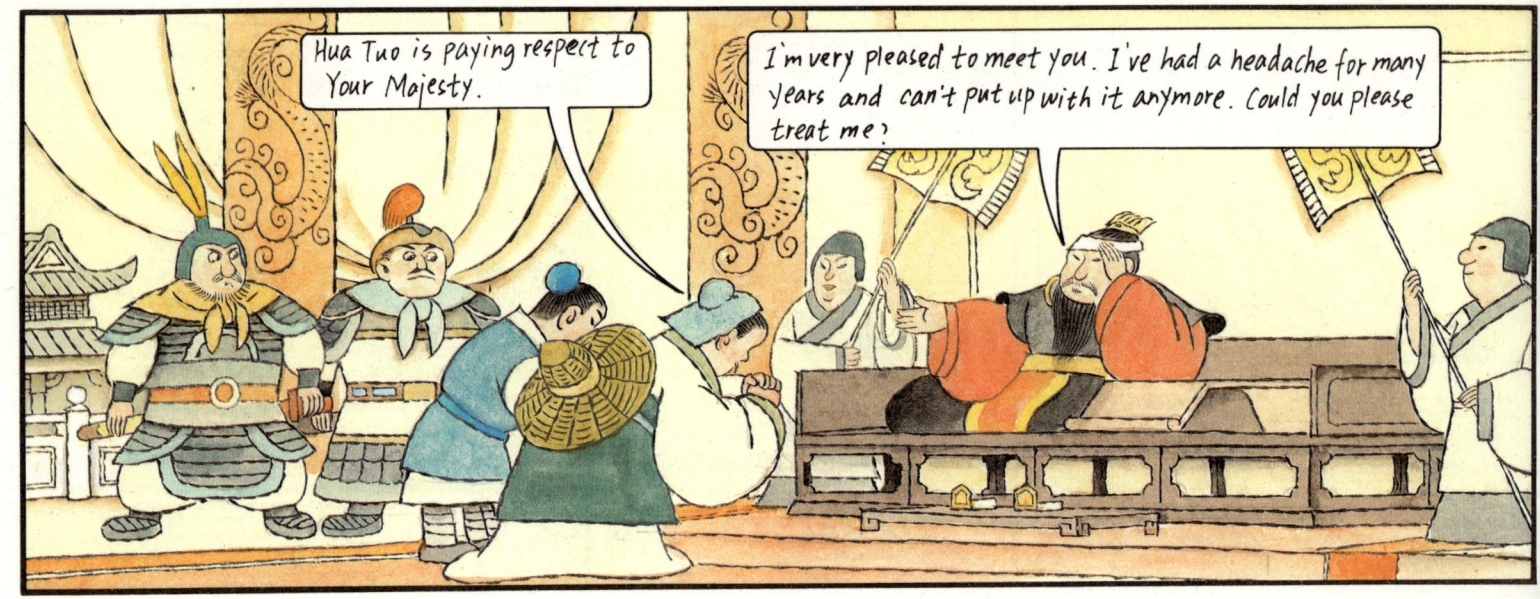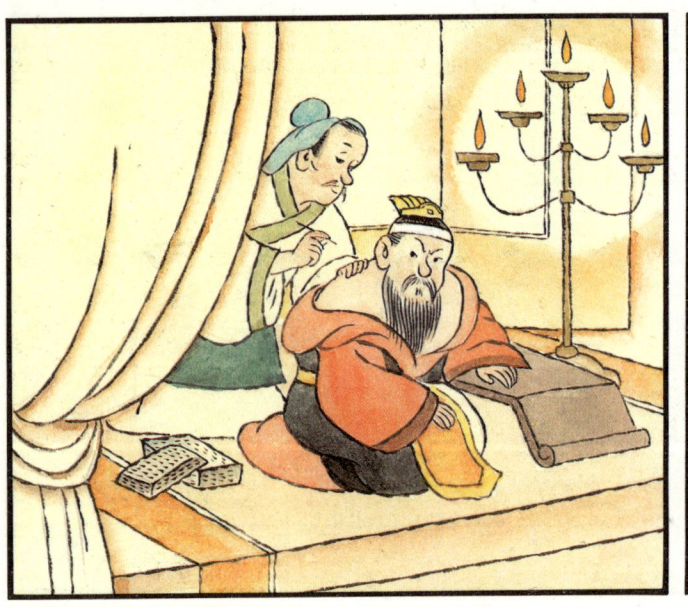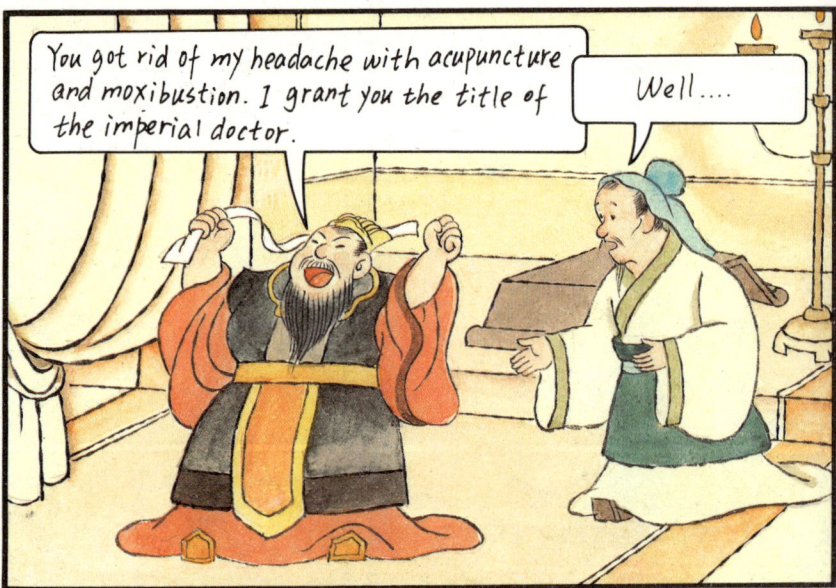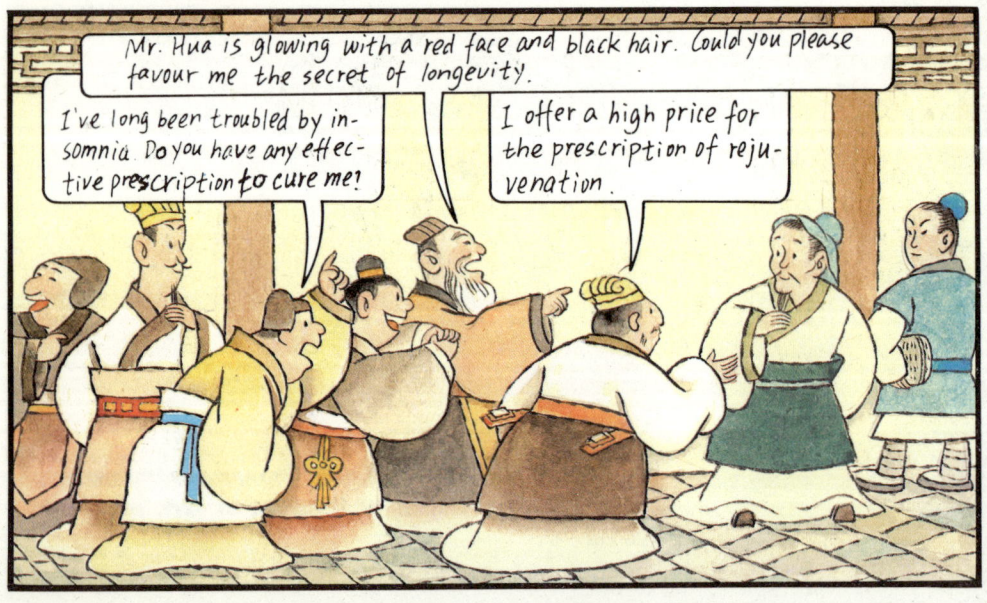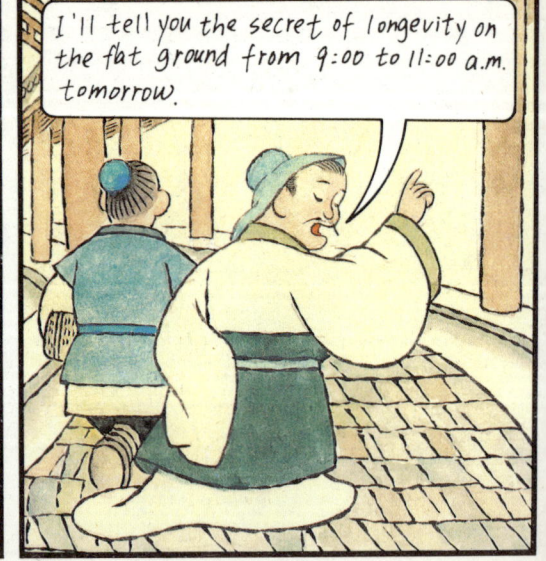

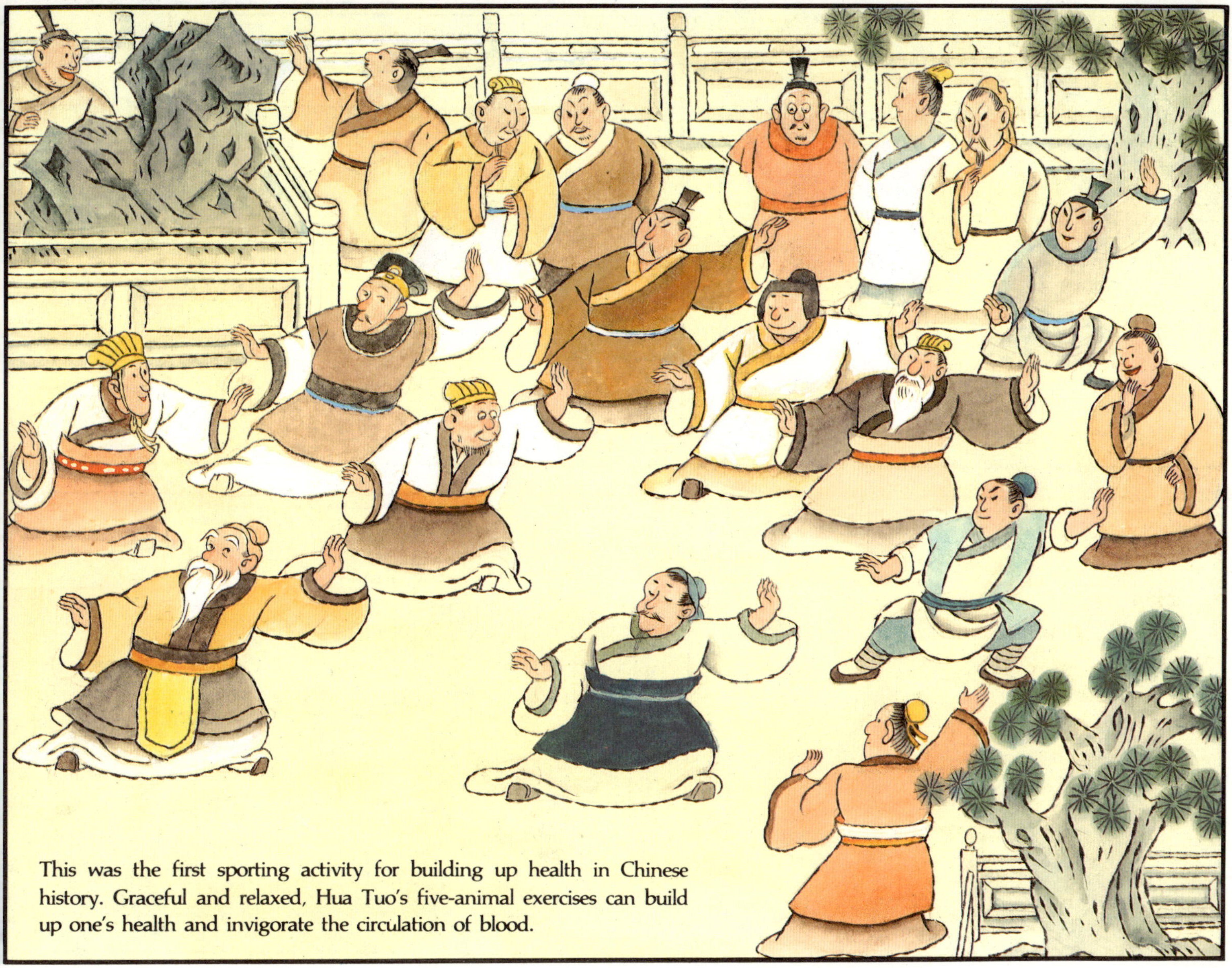

This was the first sporting activity for building up health in Chinese history. Graceful and relaxed, Hua Tuo's five-animal exercises can build up one's health and invigorate the circulation of blood.

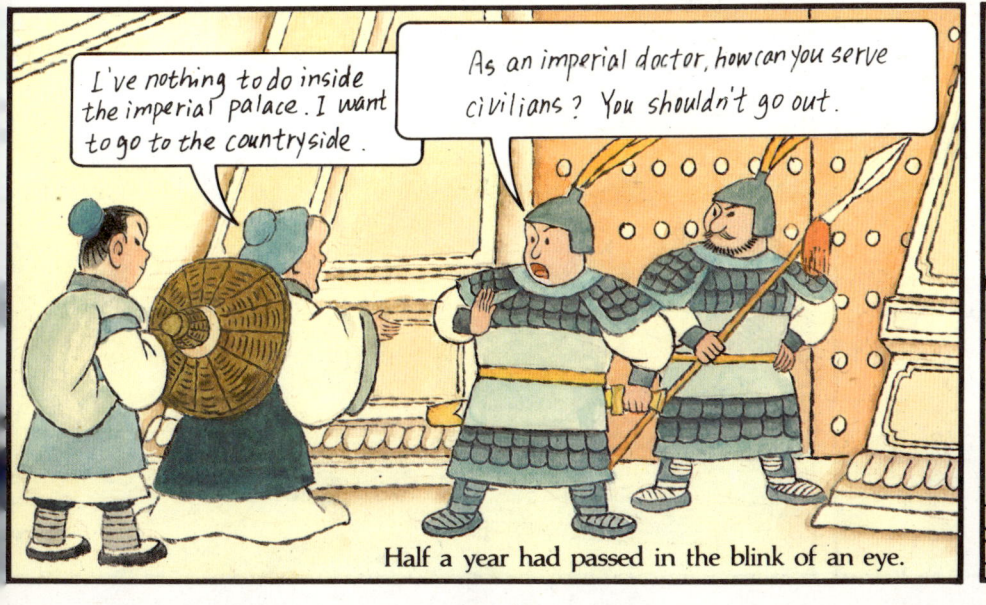

"I've nothing to do inside the imperial palace. I want to go to the countryside."

"As an imperial doctor, how can you serve civilians? You shouldn't go out."

Half a year had passed in the blink of an eye.

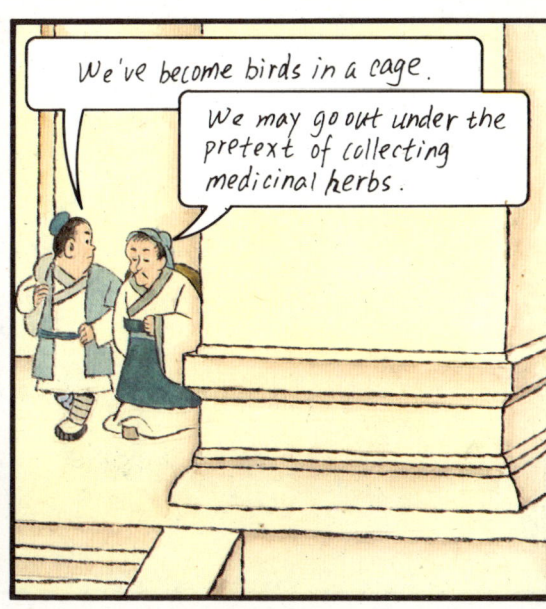

"We've become birds in a cage."

"We may go out under the pretext of collecting medicinal herbs."

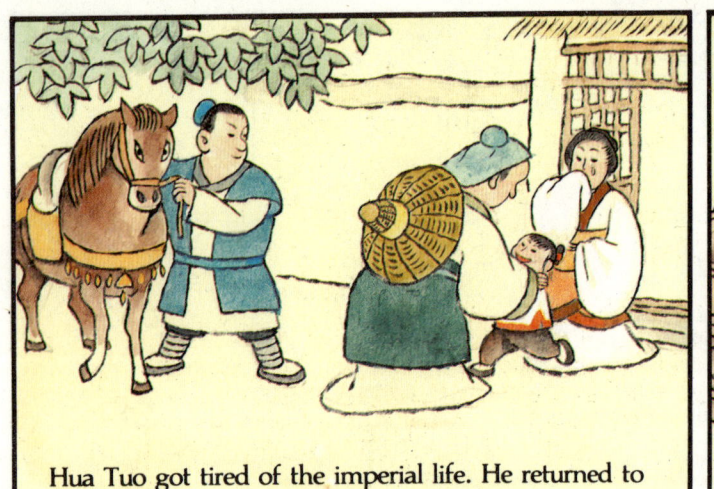
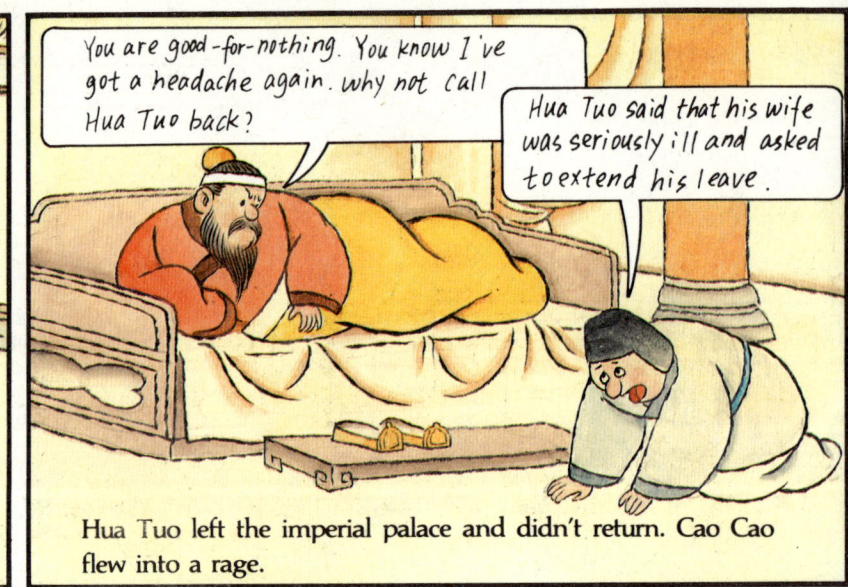

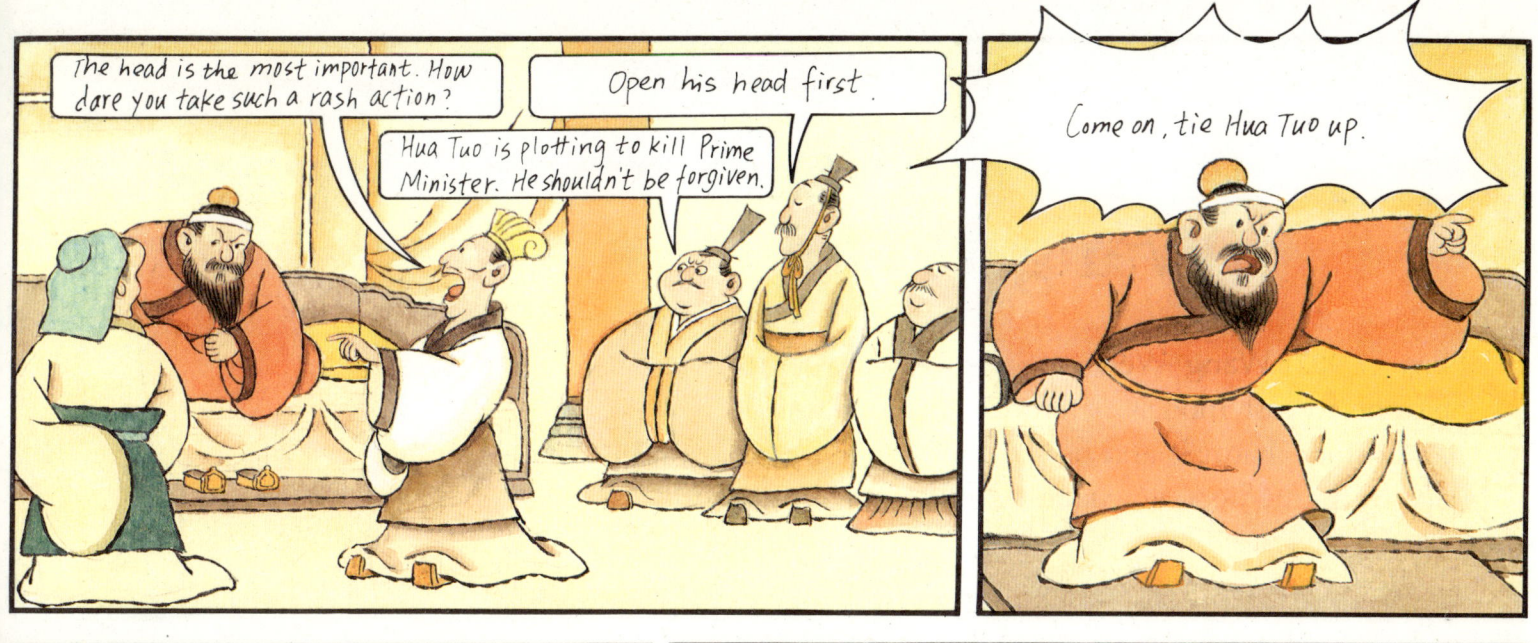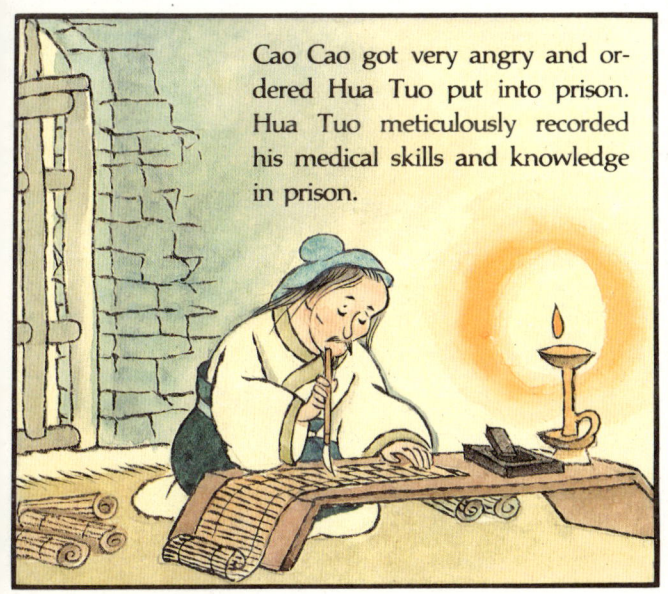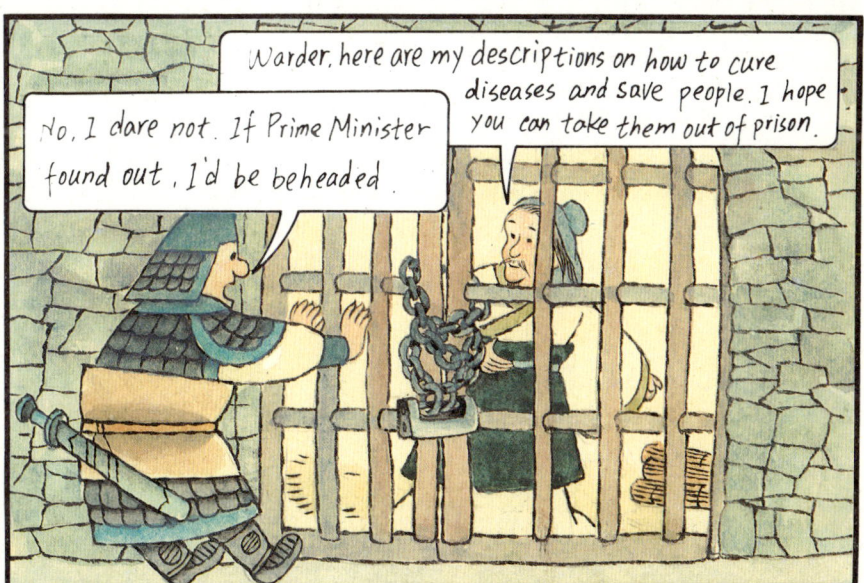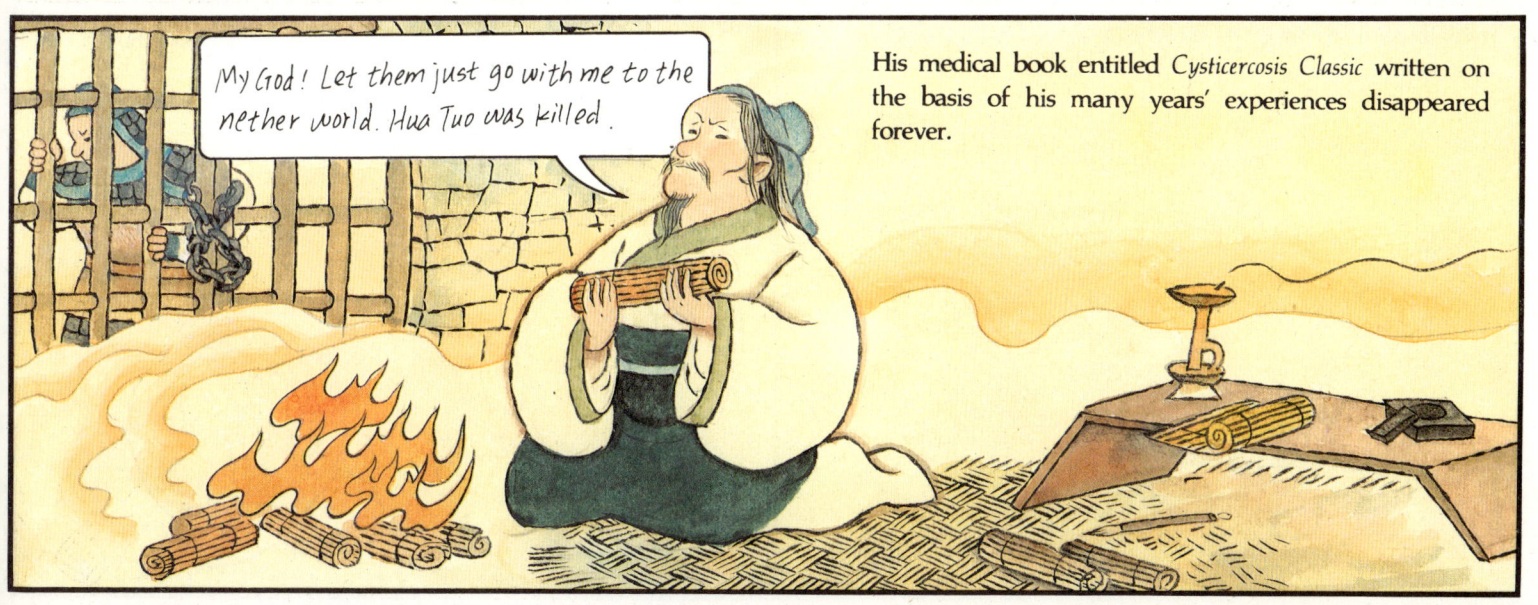

Wang Weiyi

Born in 987, Wang Weiyi, a Song Dynasty doctor, was the first one to cast models of bronze figures inscribed with the acupuncture channels and points, thus making great contributions to the traditional acupuncture and moxibustion.

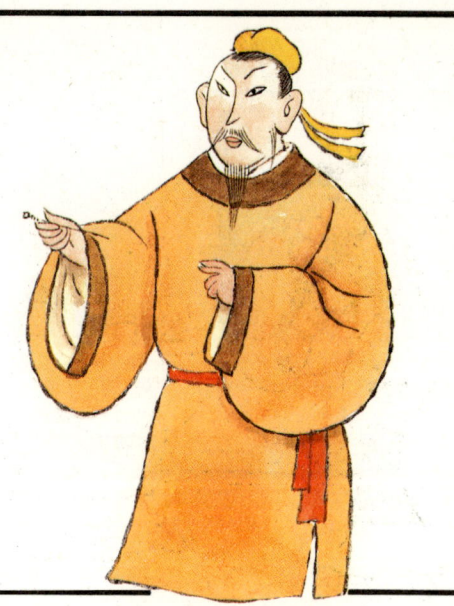

Traditional Chinese medicine held that the meridians and collaterals were pathways in which blood and *qi* (vital energy) of the human body were circulated. They formed a network and linked the tissues and organs into an organic whole. If they were impeded, a person would get a disease.

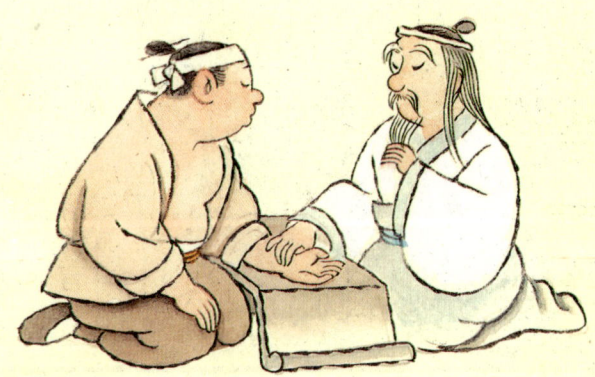

Acupuncture therapy — puncturing a silver needle in a certain location of the meridians, twisting, turning, lifting and inserting the needle to cure the disease by means of clearing the meridians.

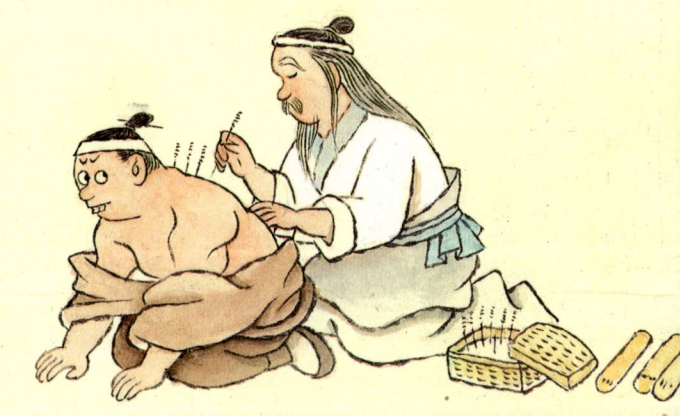

Moxibustion therapy — scorching acupoints with lighting moxa.

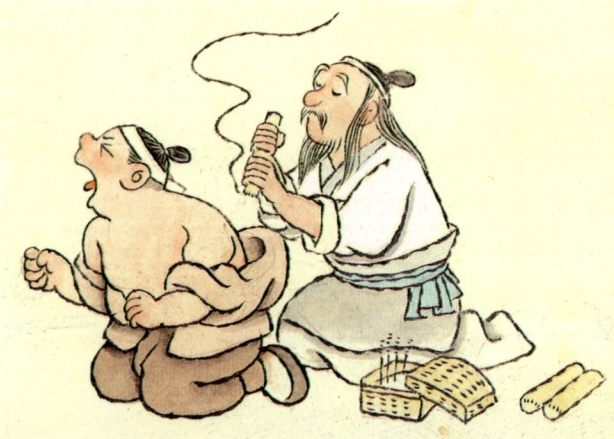

The unique acupuncture and moxibustion therapy has a history of at least 2,500 years in China.

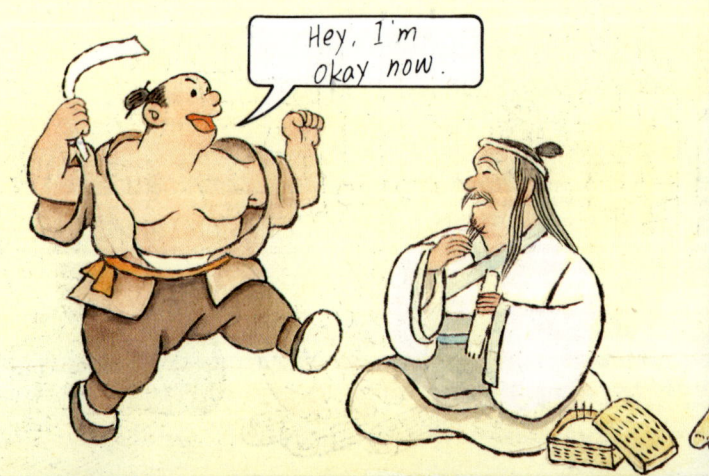

"Hey, I'm okay now."

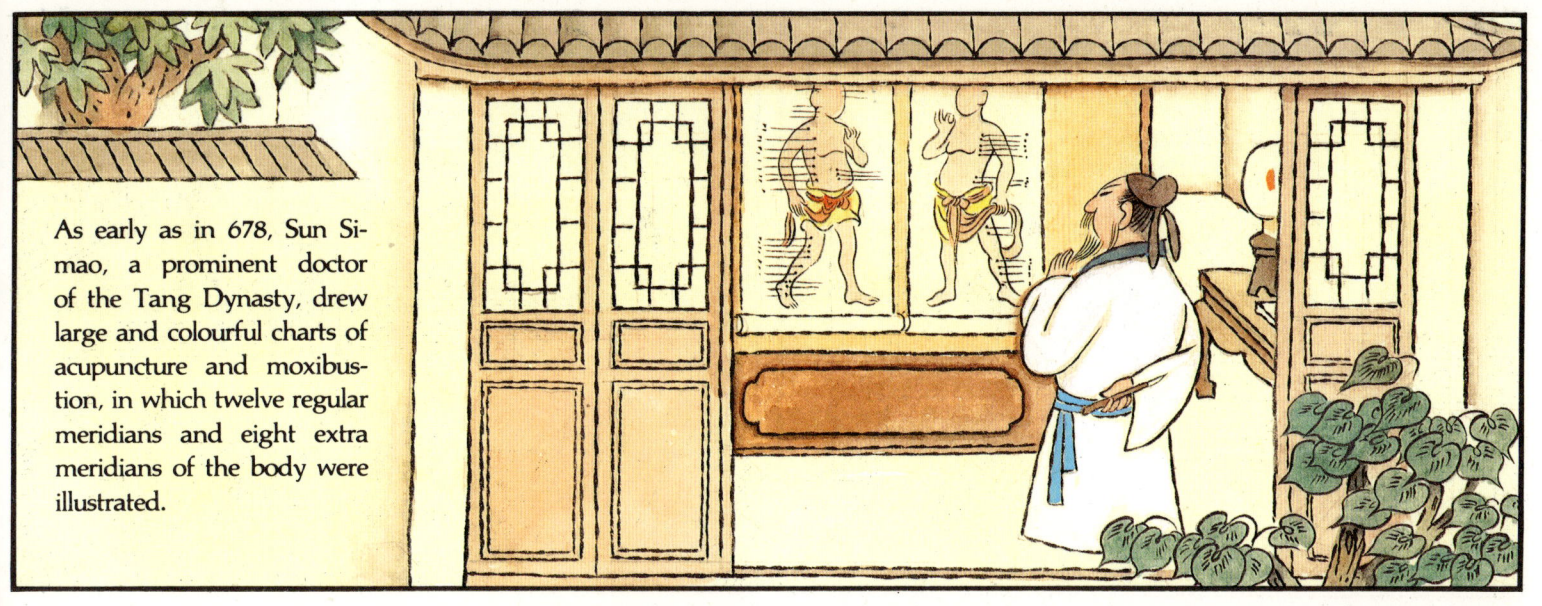

As early as in 678, Sun Si-mao, a prominent doctor of the Tang Dynasty, drew large and colourful charts of acupuncture and moxibustion, in which twelve regular meridians and eight extra meridians of the body were illustrated.

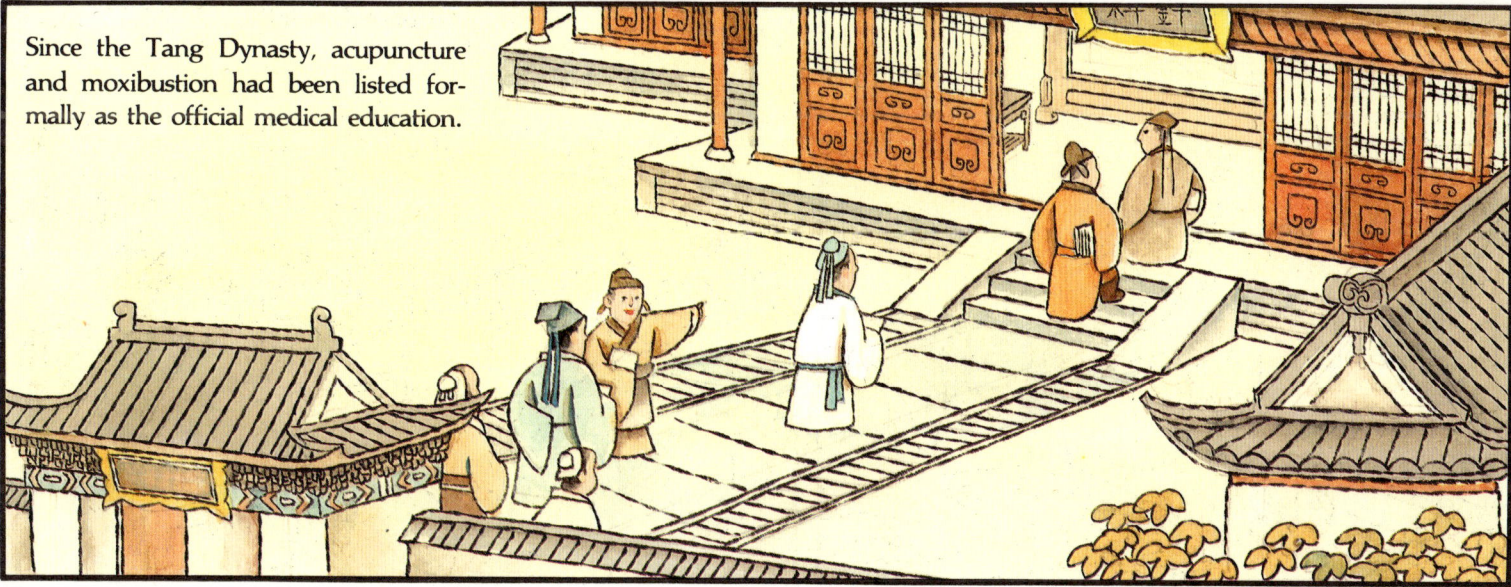

Since the Tang Dynasty, acupuncture and moxibustion had been listed formally as the official medical education.

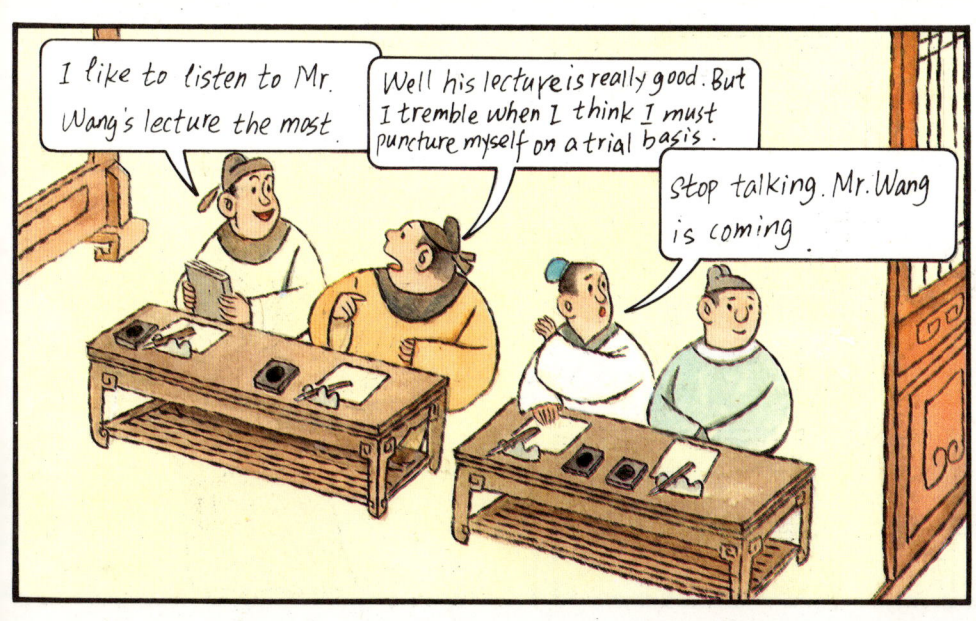
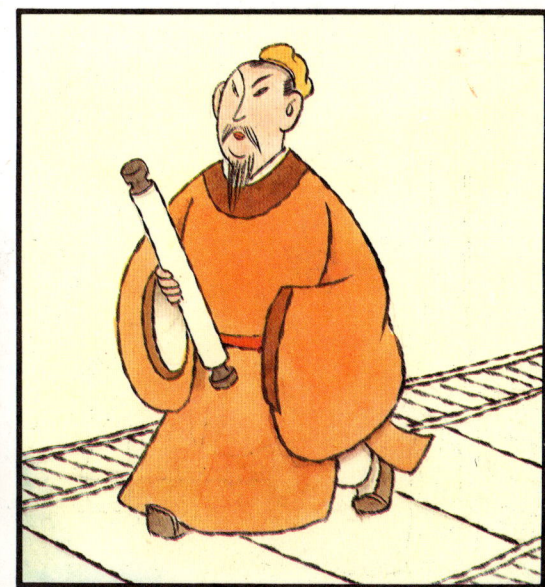

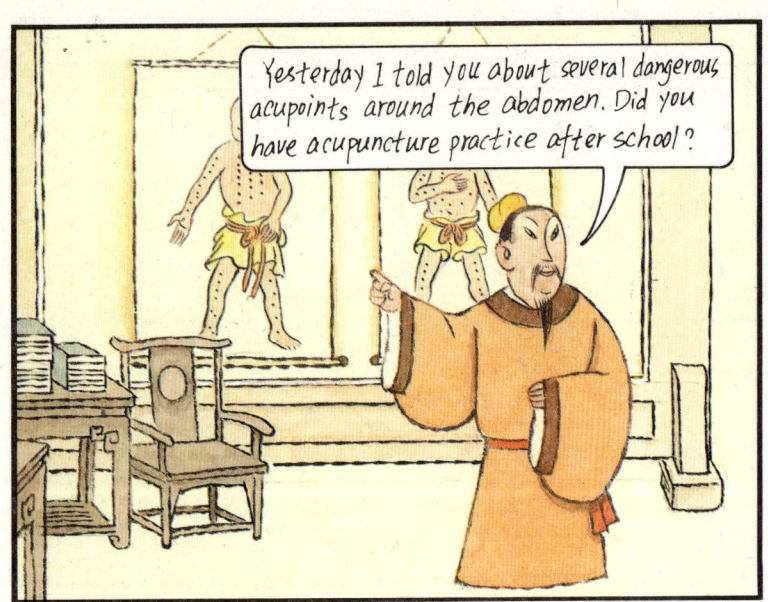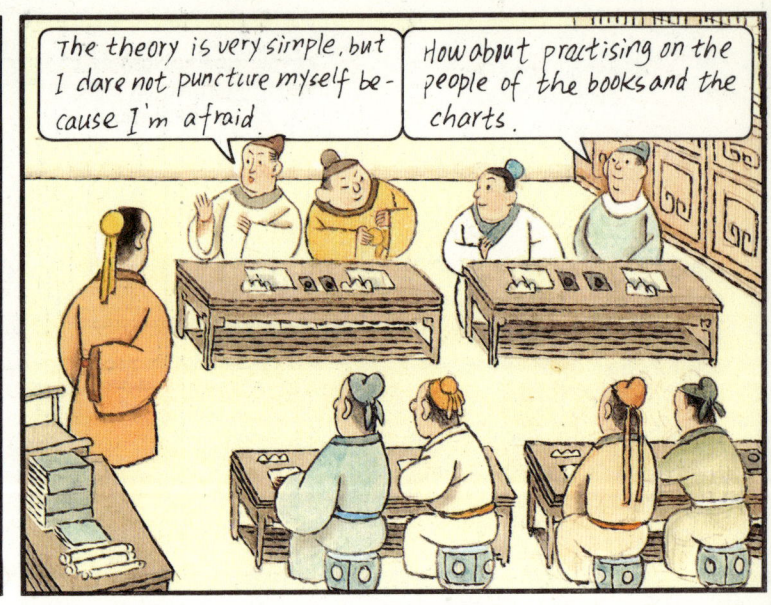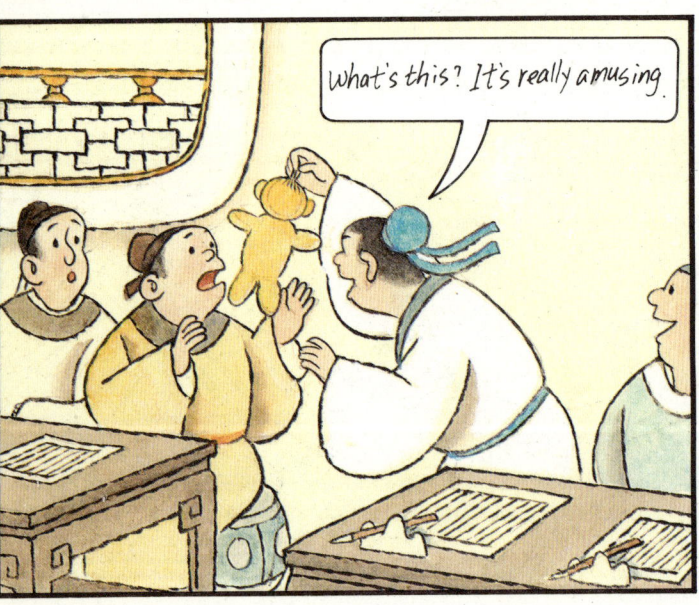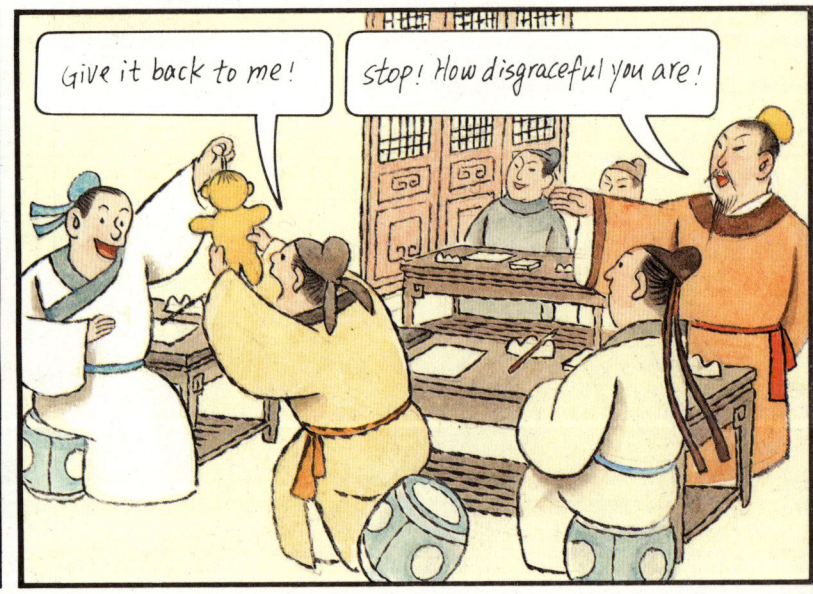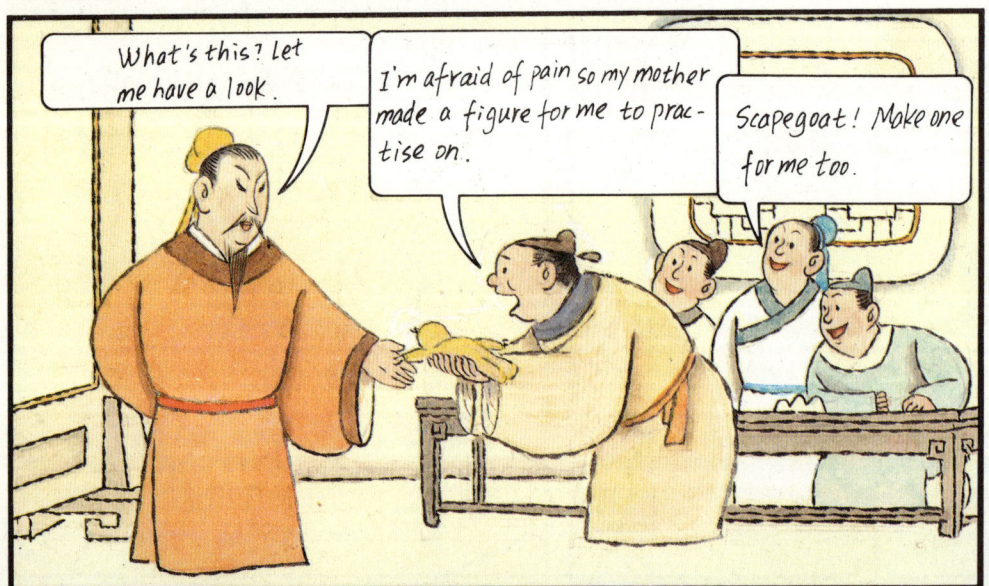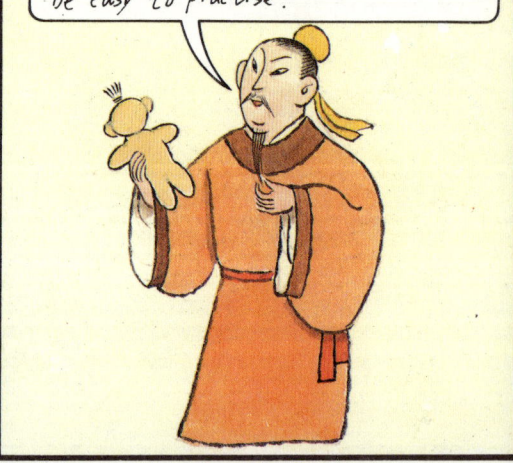

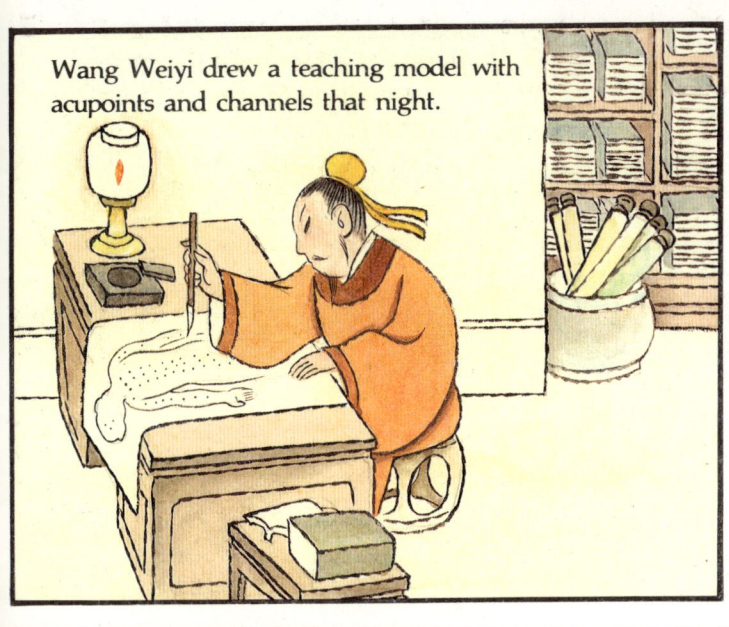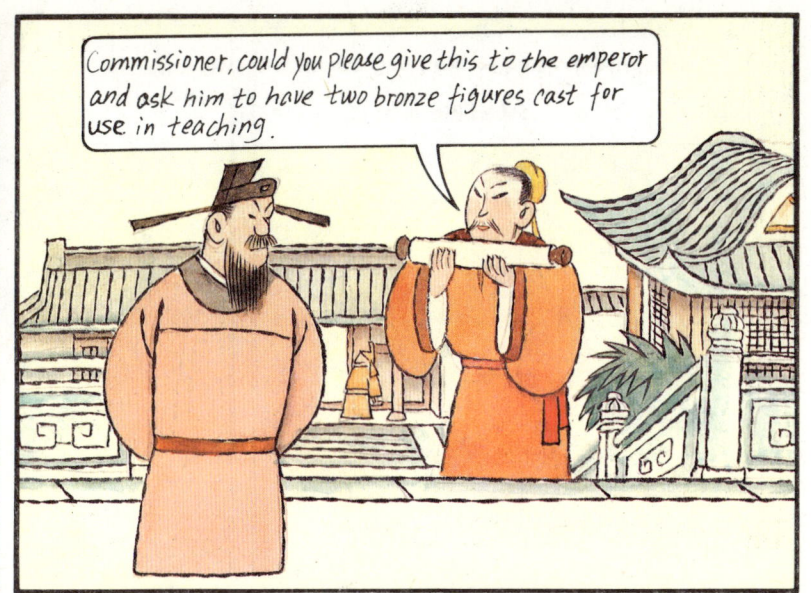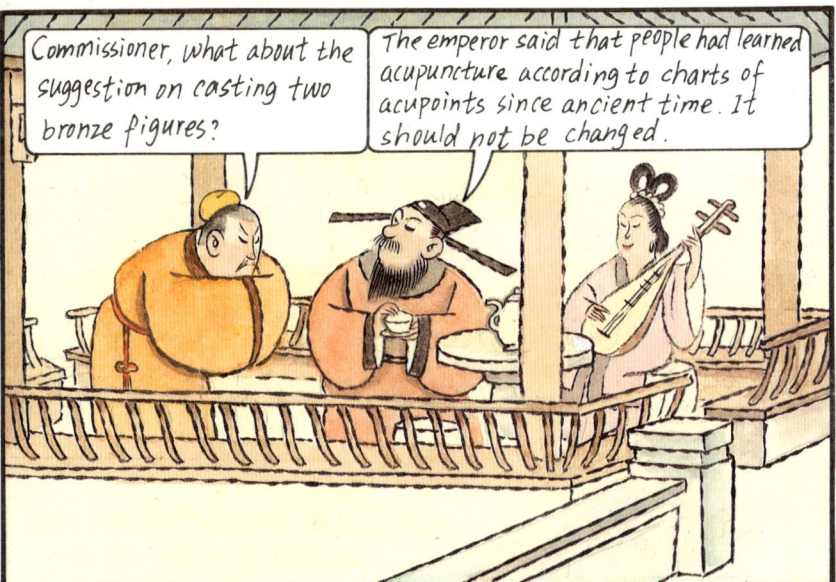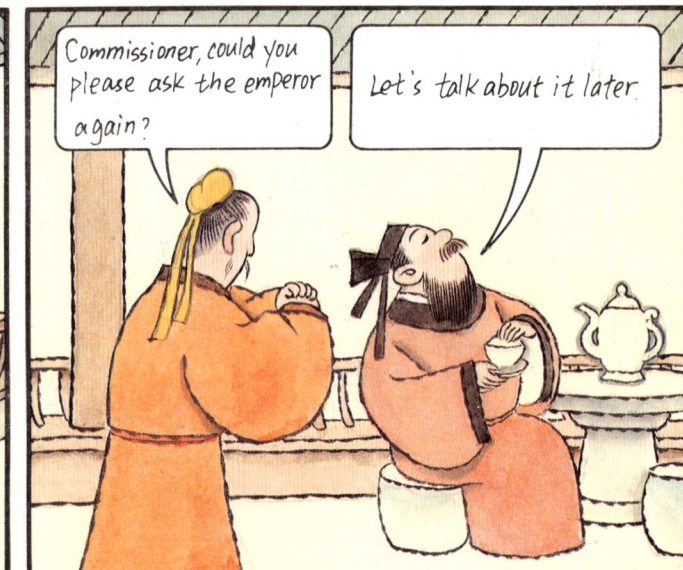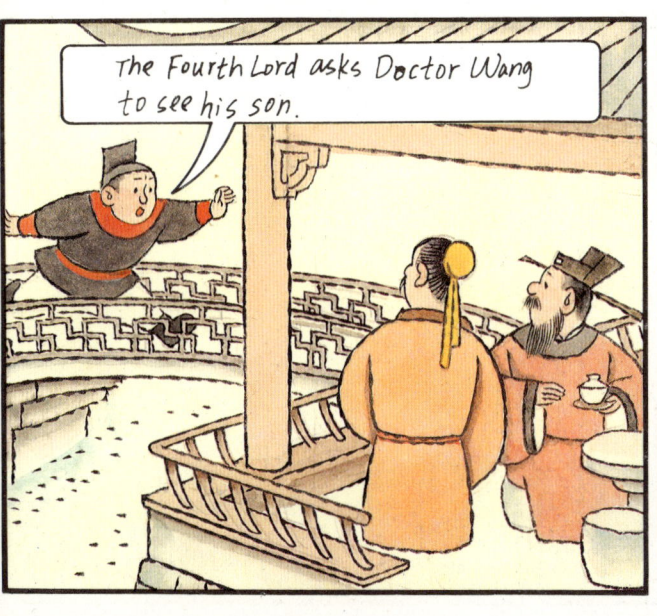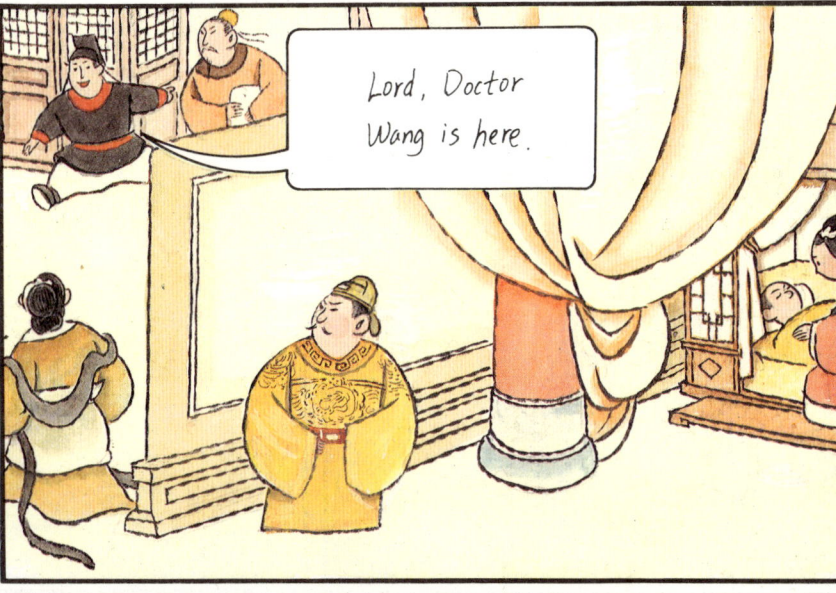

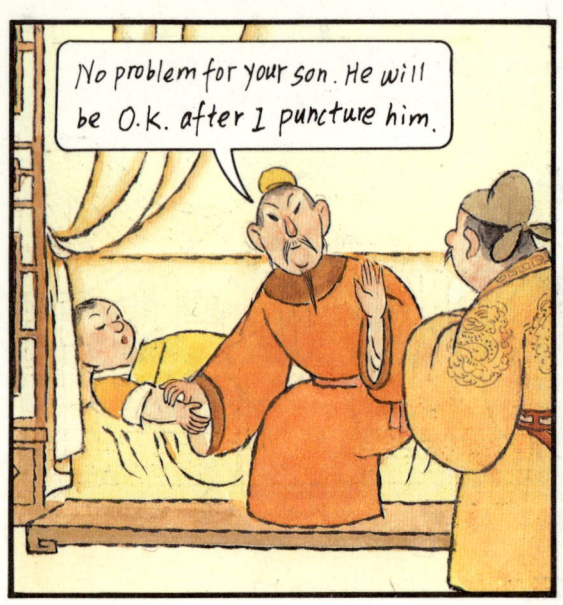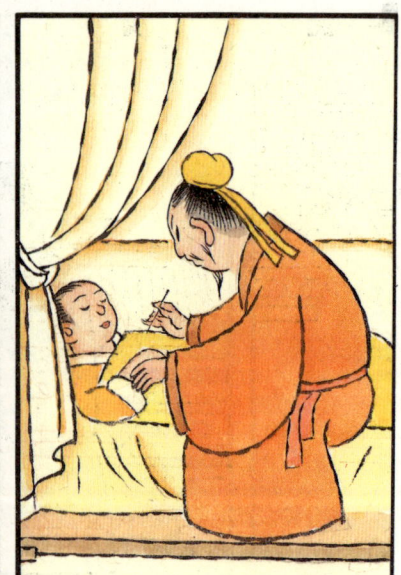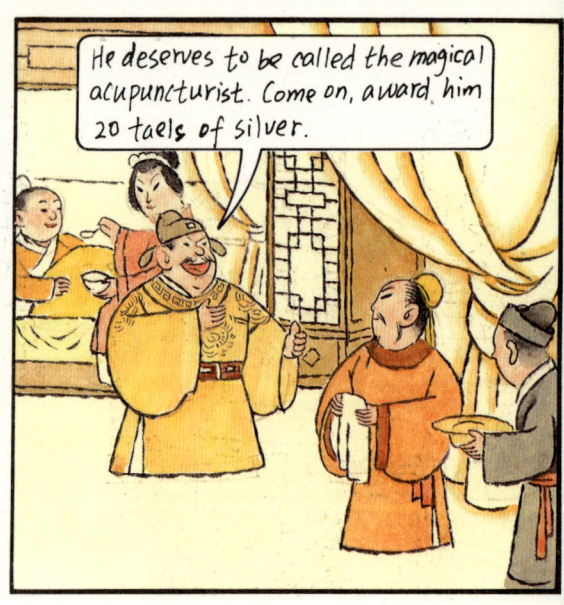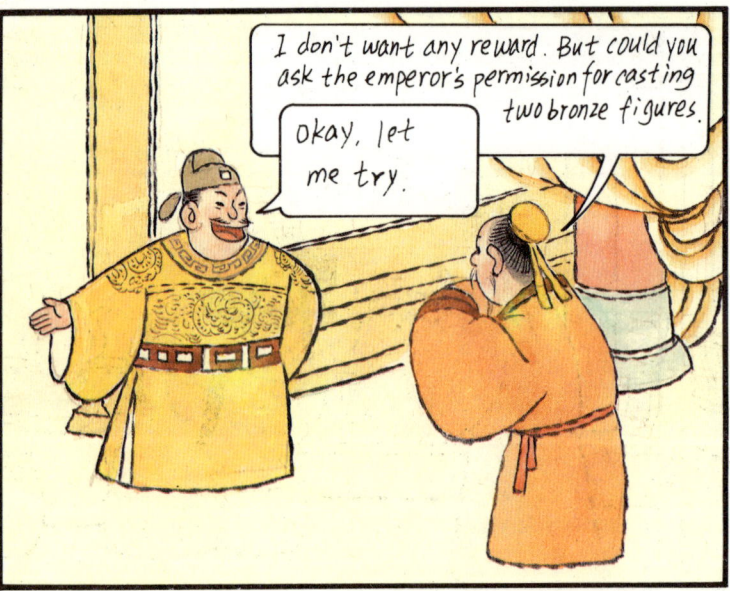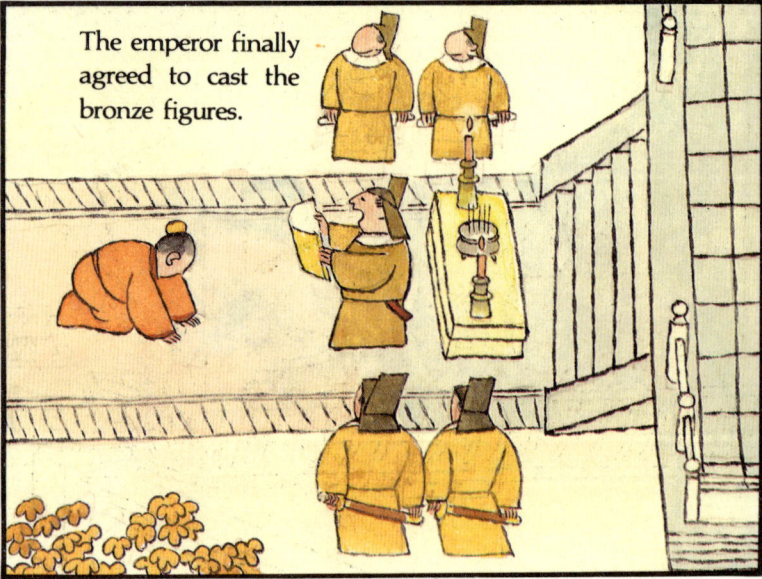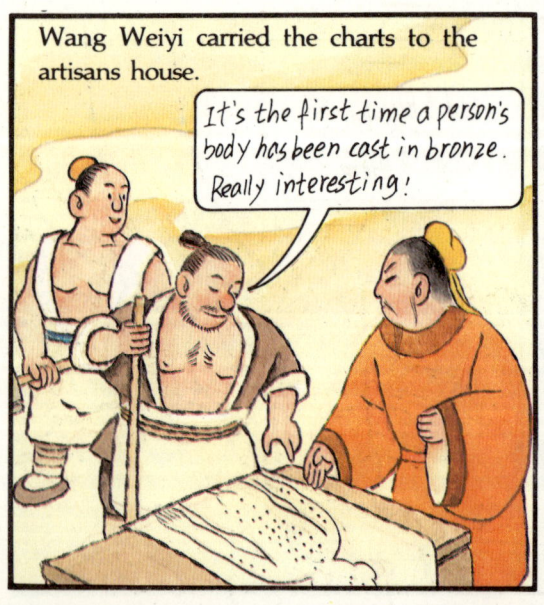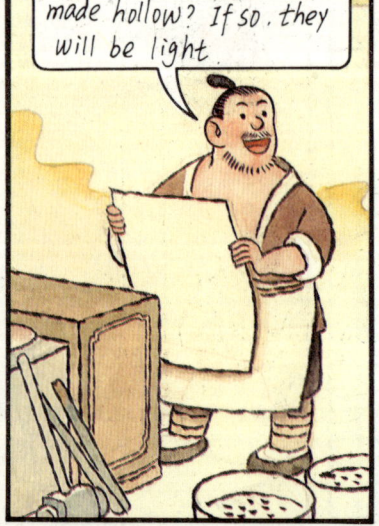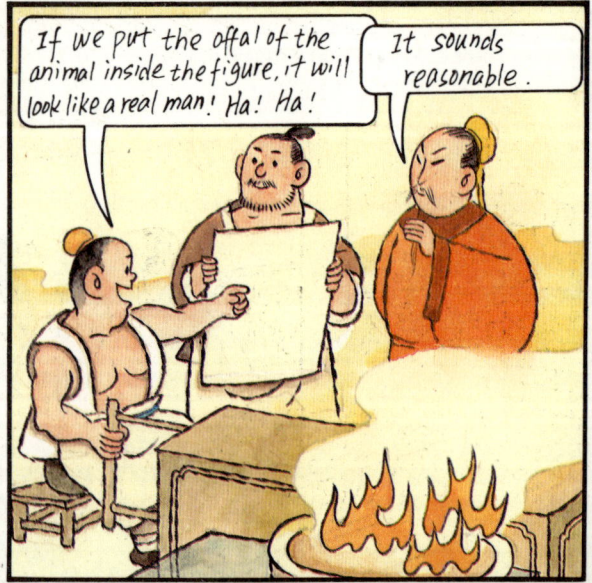

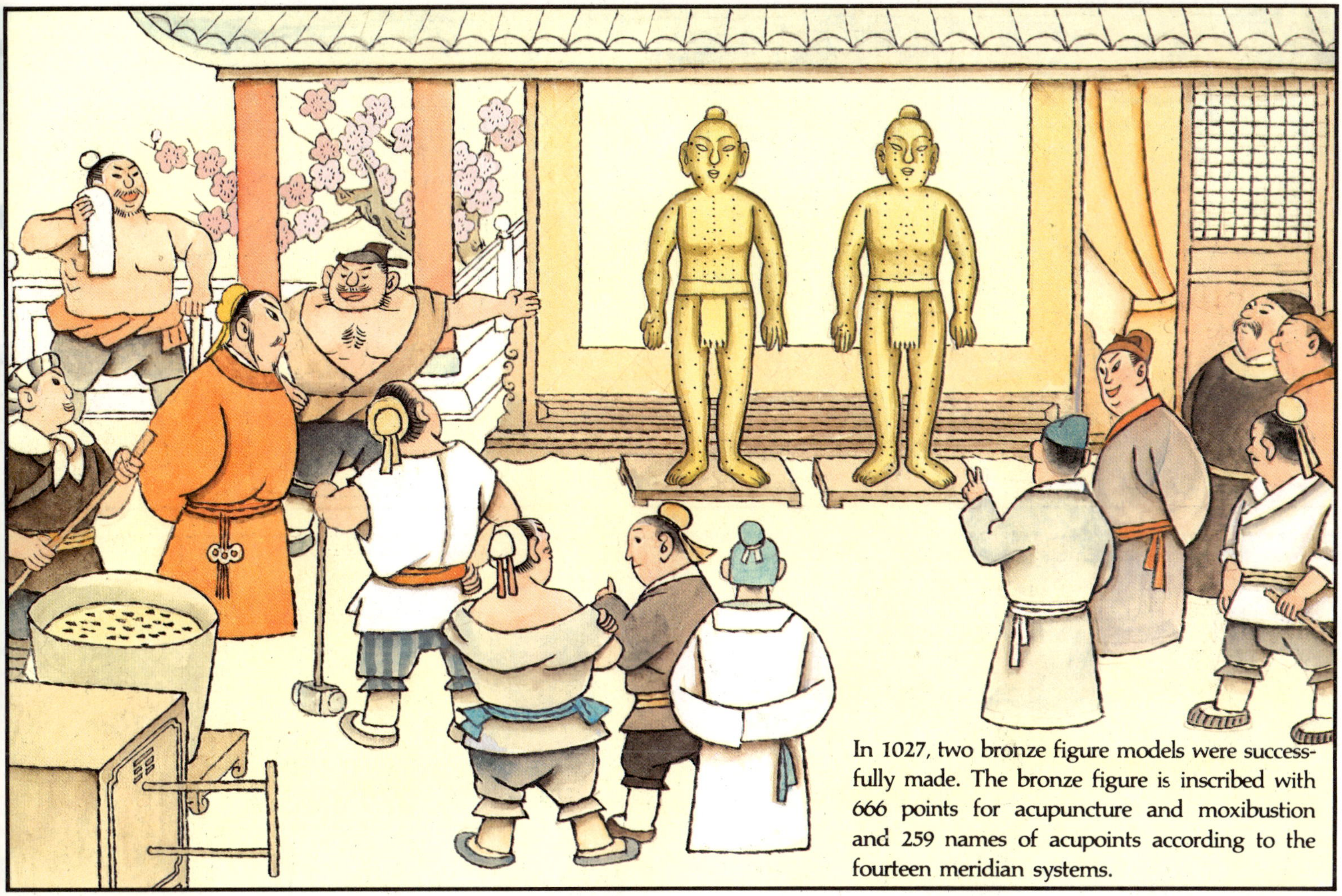

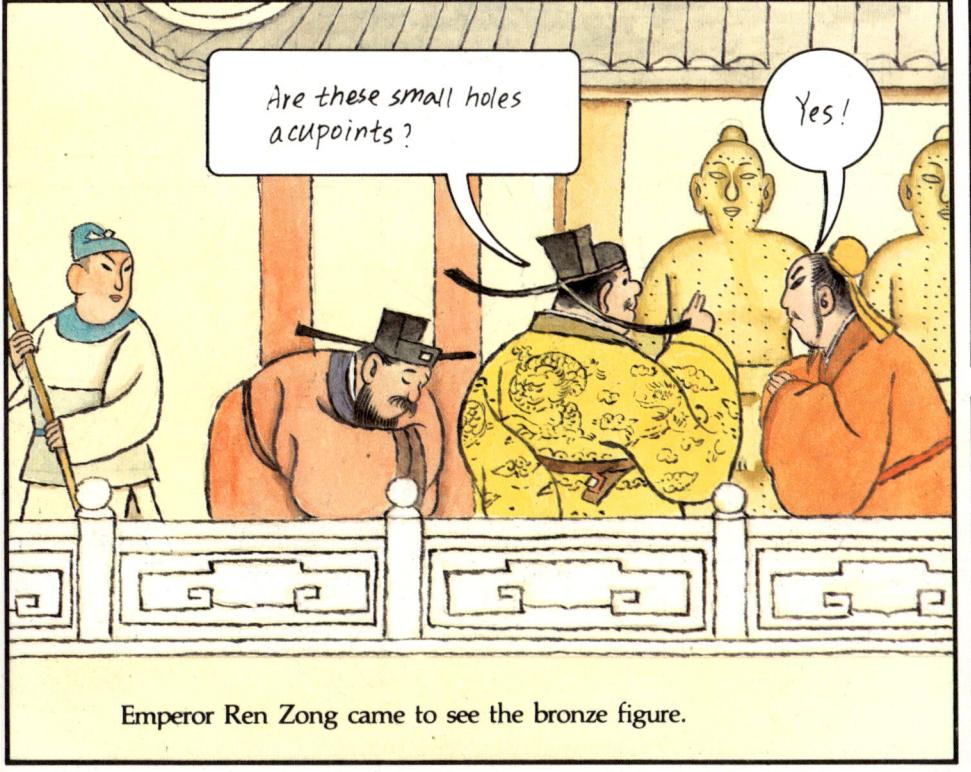

In 1027, two bronze figure models were successfully made. The bronze figure is inscribed with 666 points for acupuncture and moxibustion and 259 names of acupoints according to the fourteen meridian systems.

Emperor Ren Zong came to see the bronze figure.

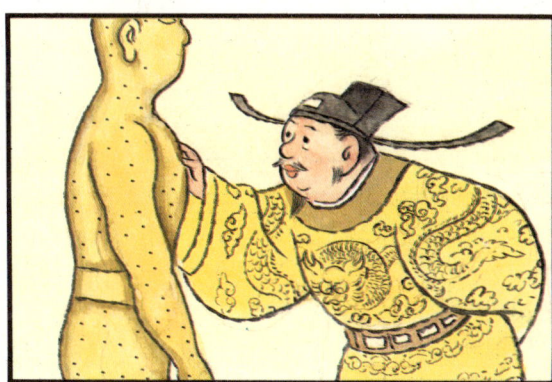

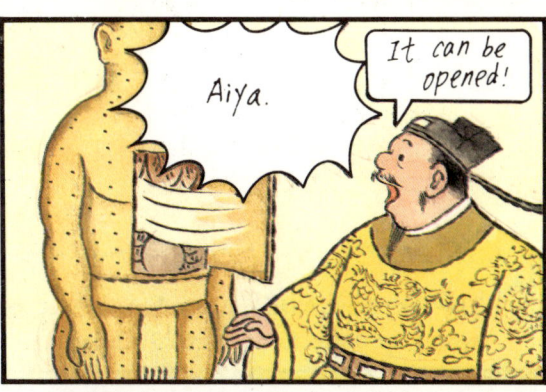

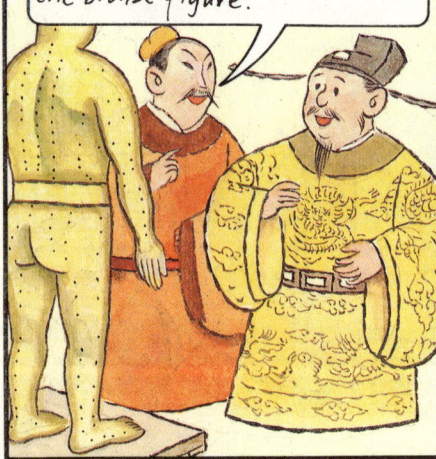
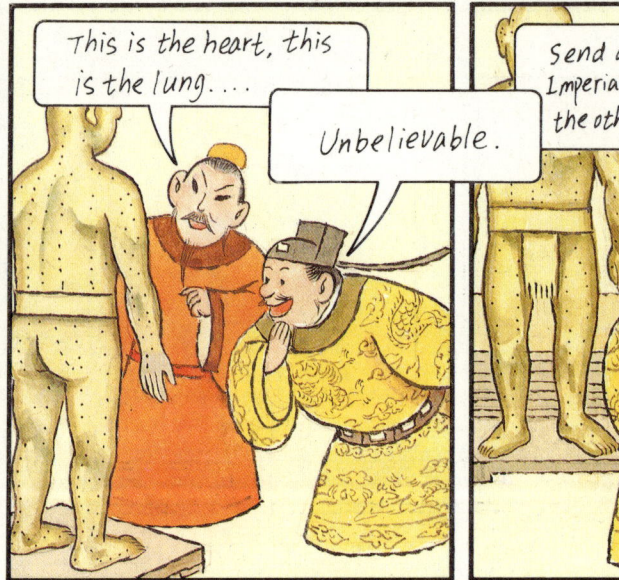
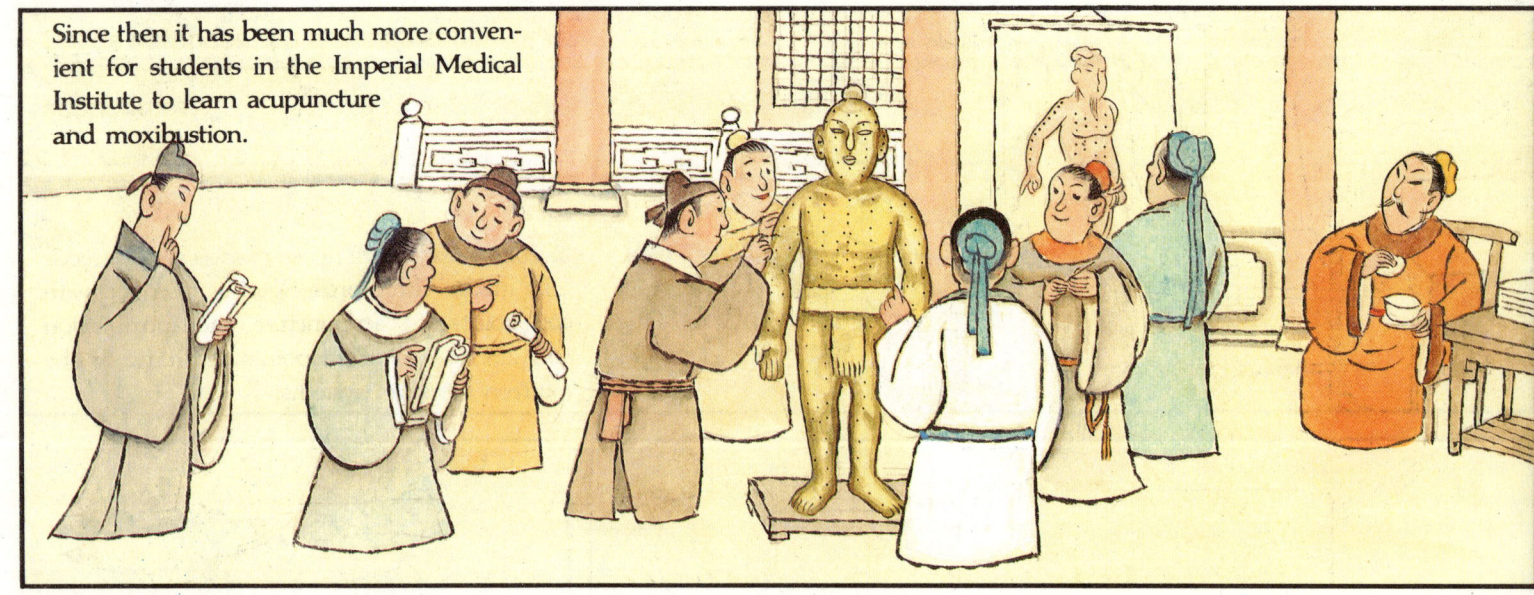
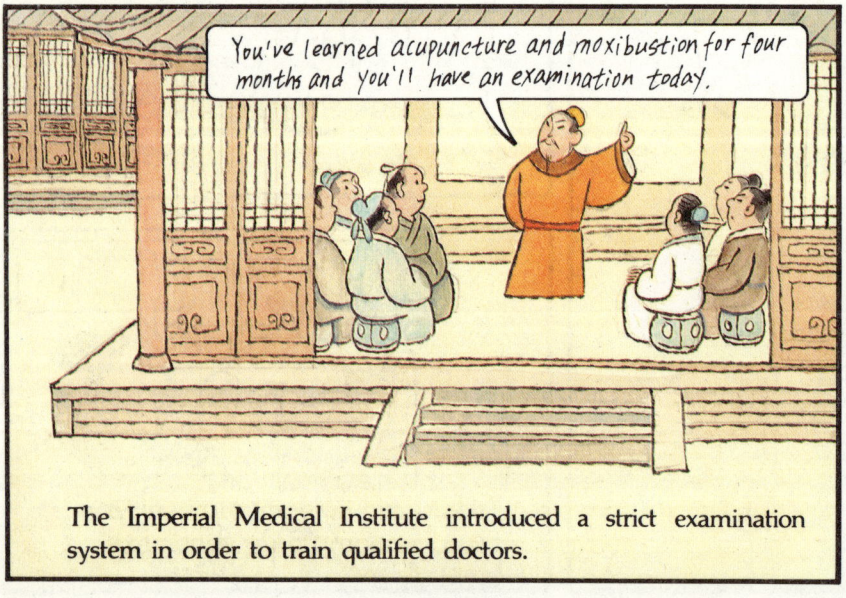
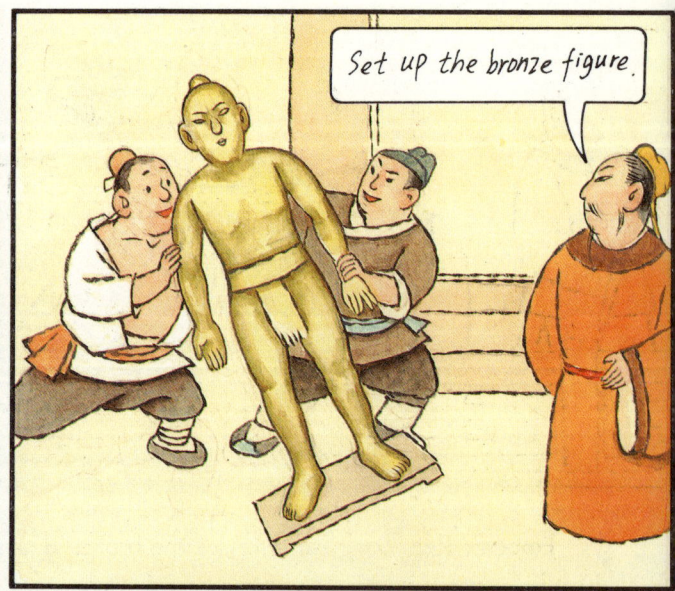

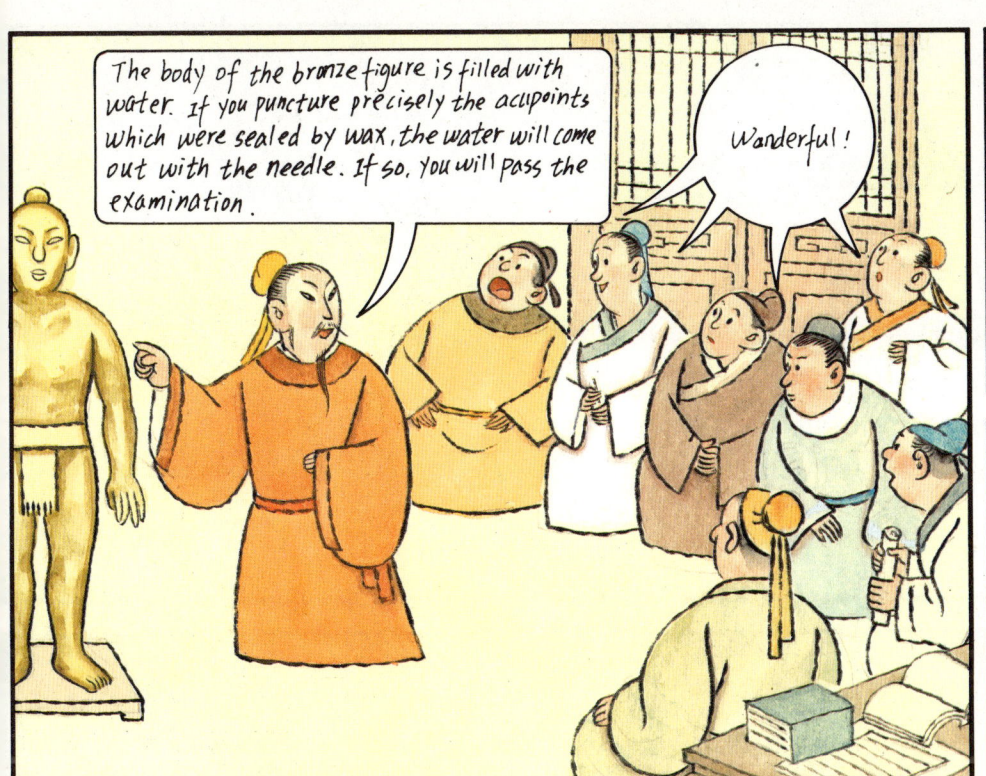
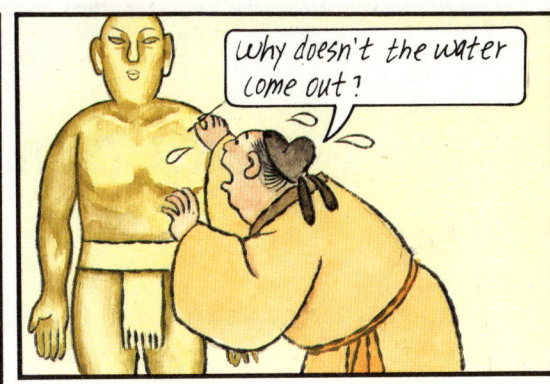
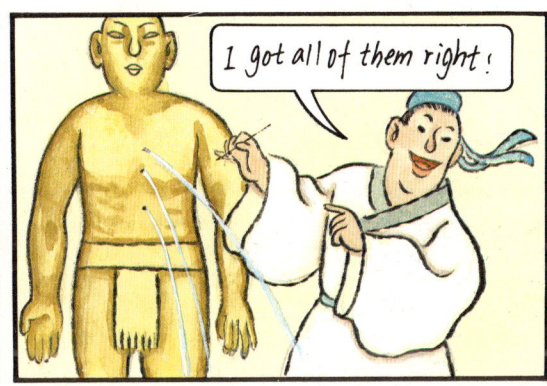
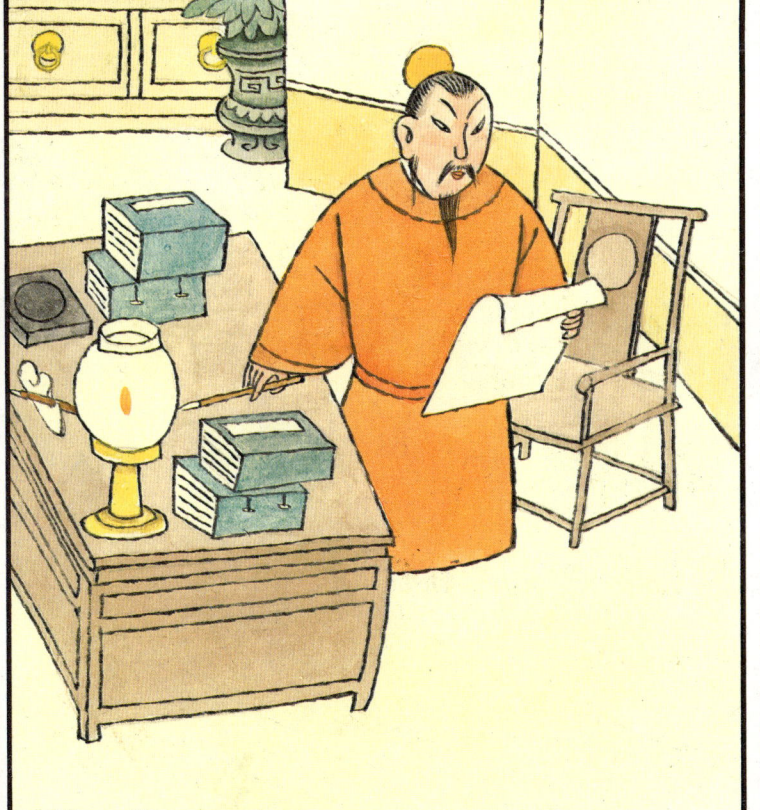

Wang Weiyi summed up acupuncture before the Song Dynasty, and corrected many mistakes. He also wrote a three-volume book entitled *Illustrated Manual of Acupoints on Bronze Figure*, which became a model for acupuncture at that time.

In the same year, the *Illustrated Manual of Acupoints* was engraved on a stone tablet so more people could learn about it.

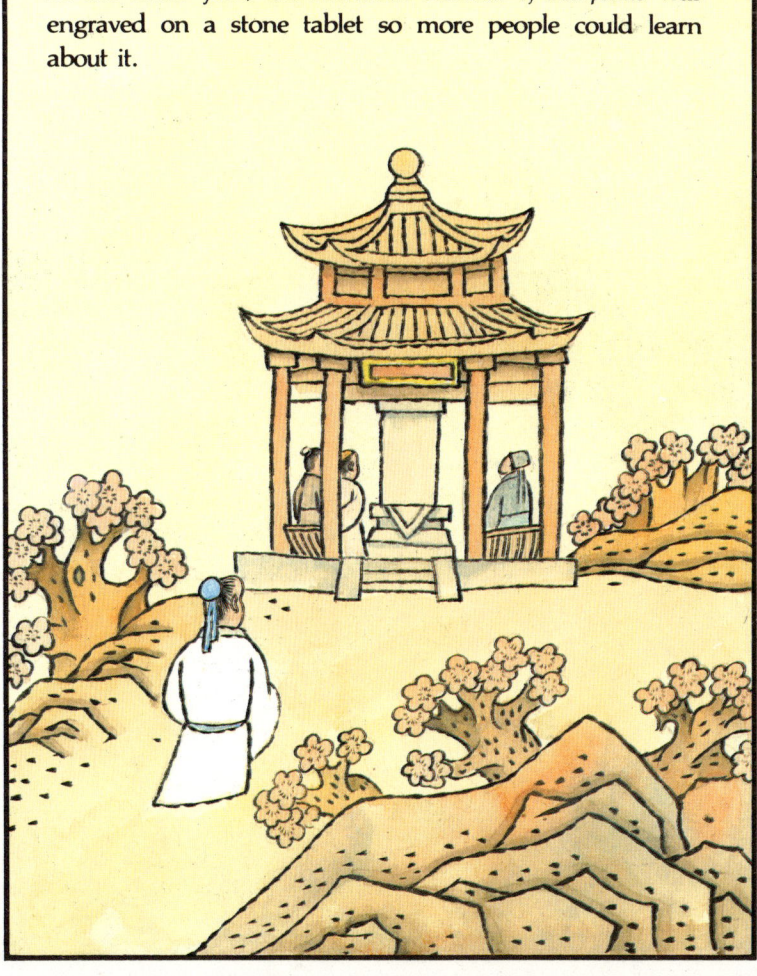

Li Shizhen

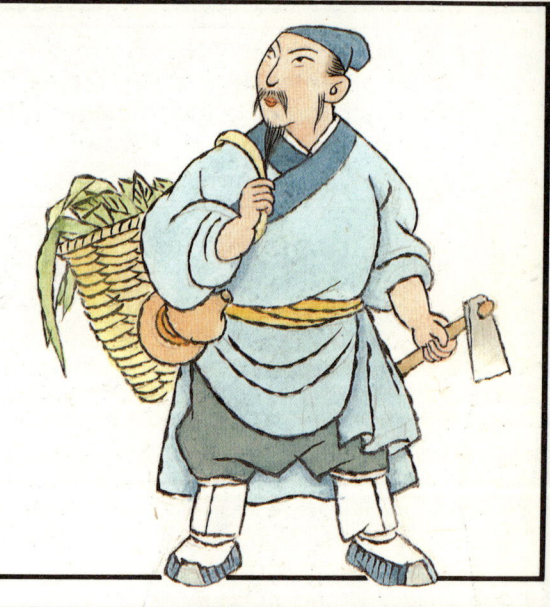

Li Shizhen (1518–1593) was a distinguished doctor of the Ming Dynasty. He spent 27 years writing the most complete guide to medicines of ancient China entitled *Compendium of Materia Medica*.

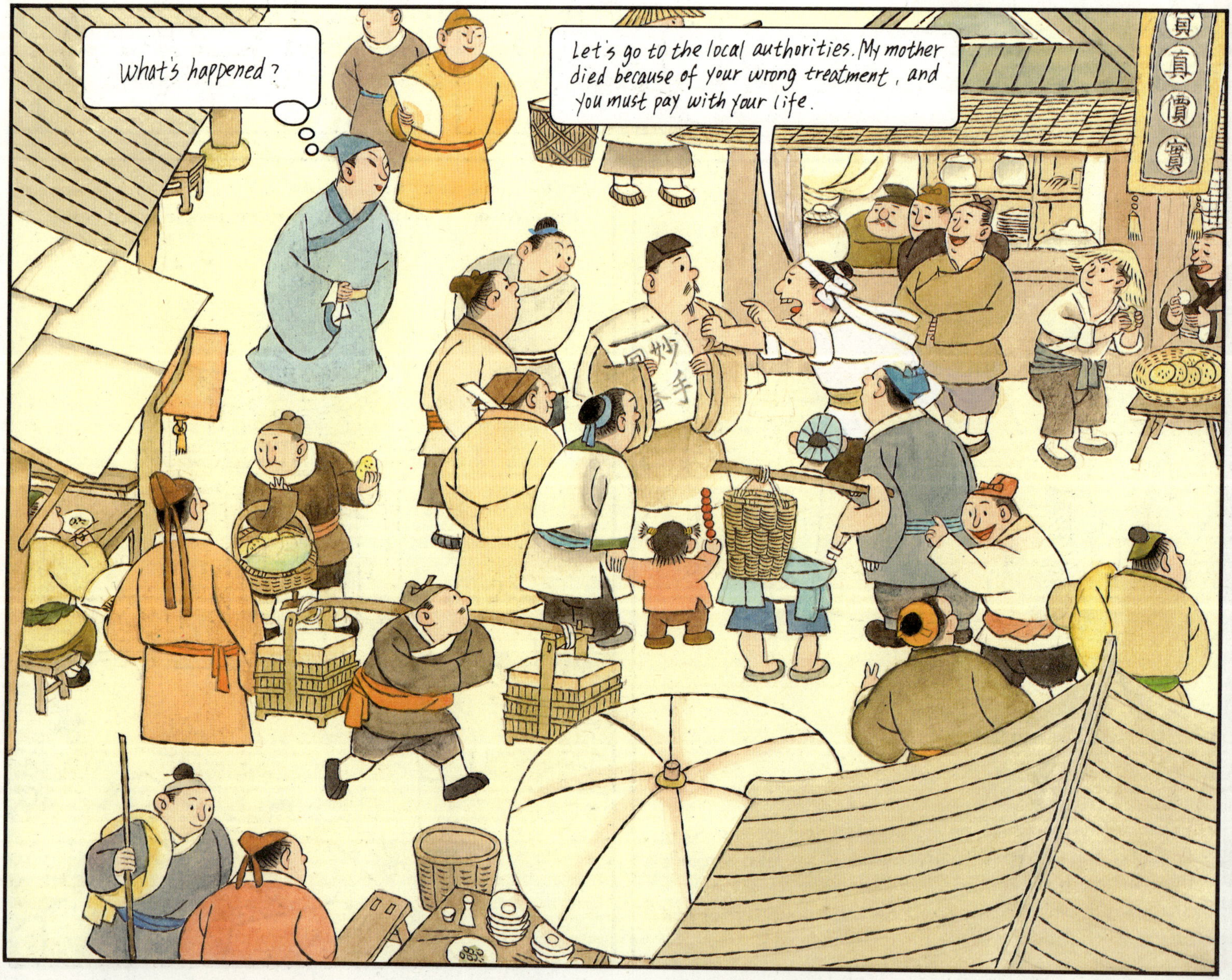

> What's happened?

> Let's go to the local authorities. My mother died because of your wrong treatment, and you must pay with your life.

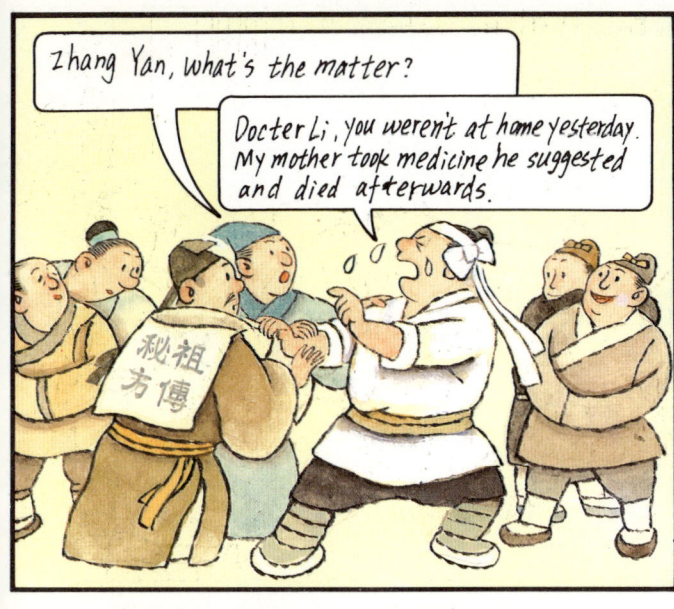
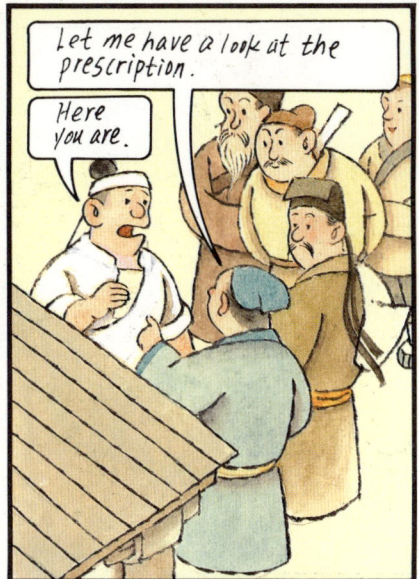
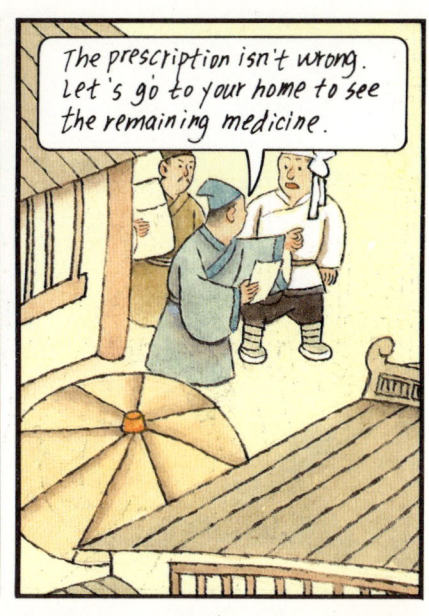
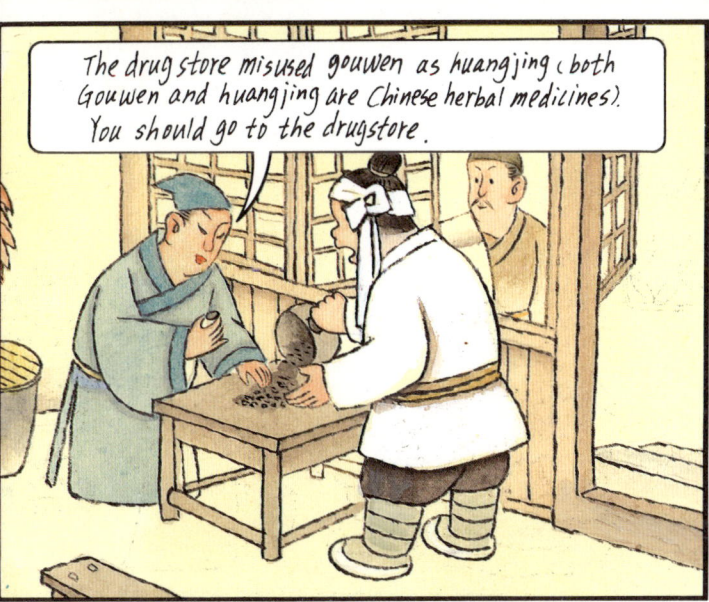
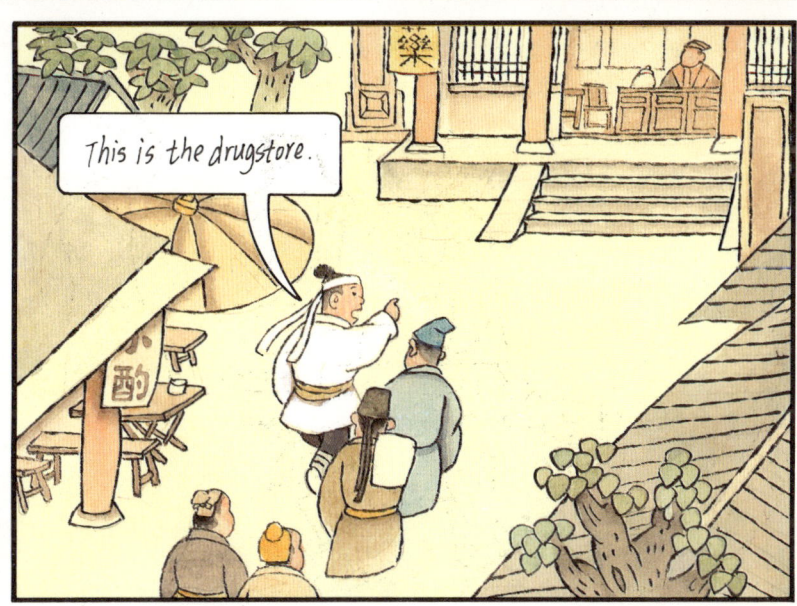
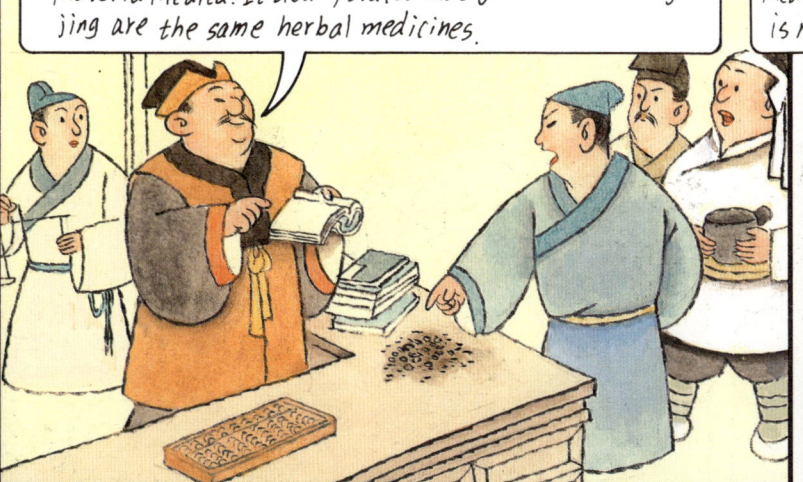
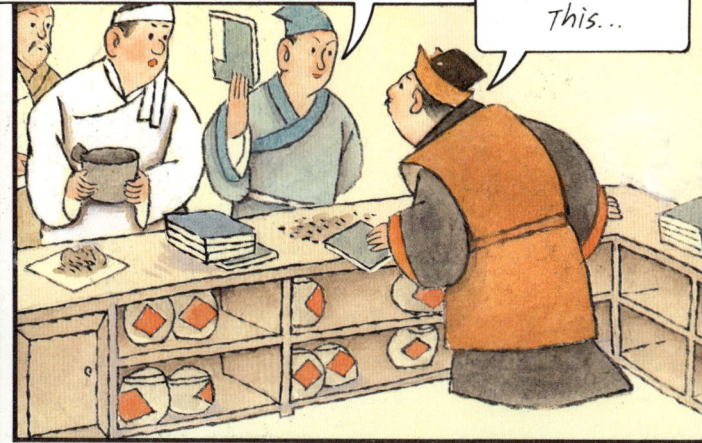

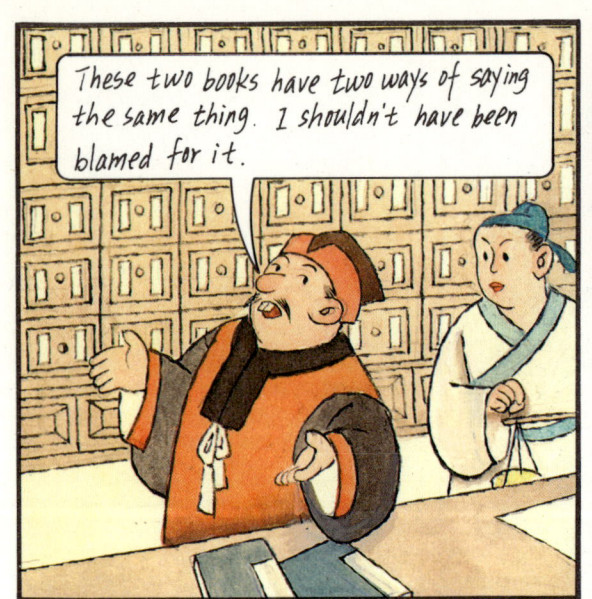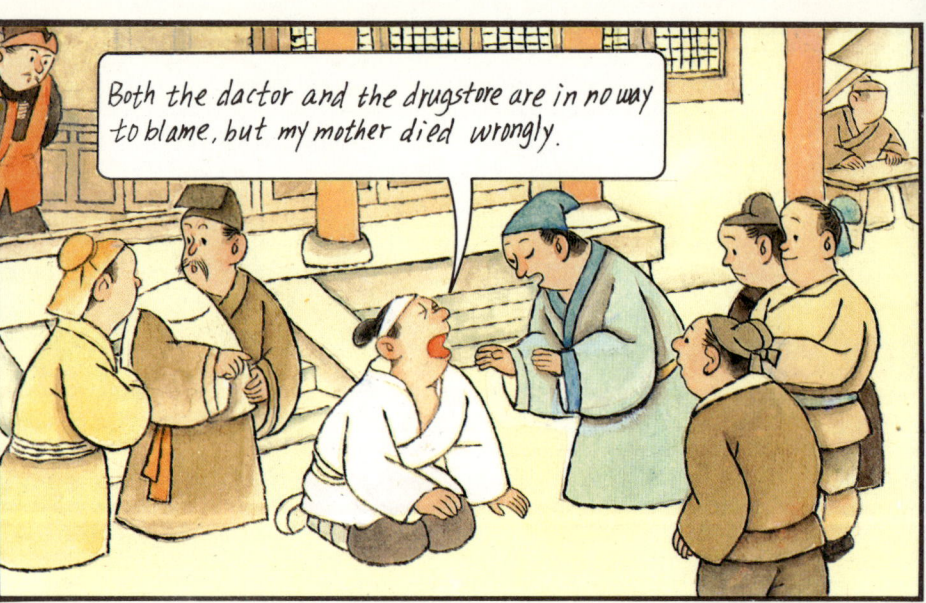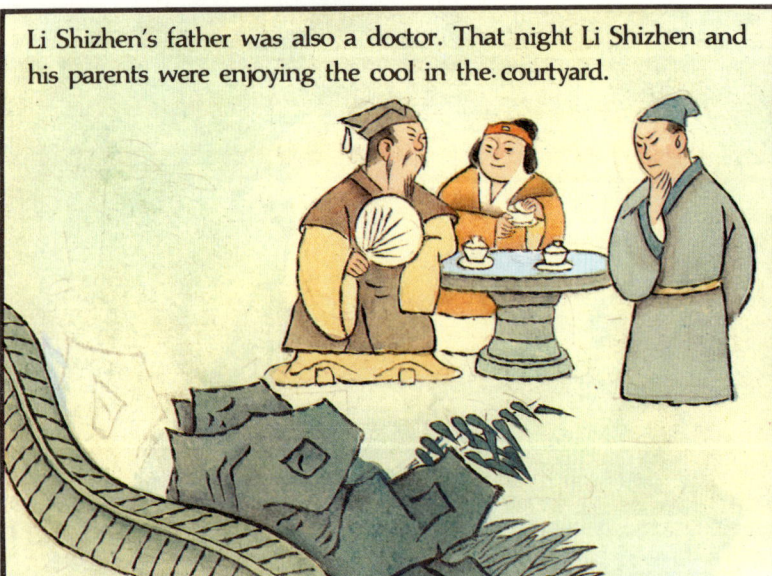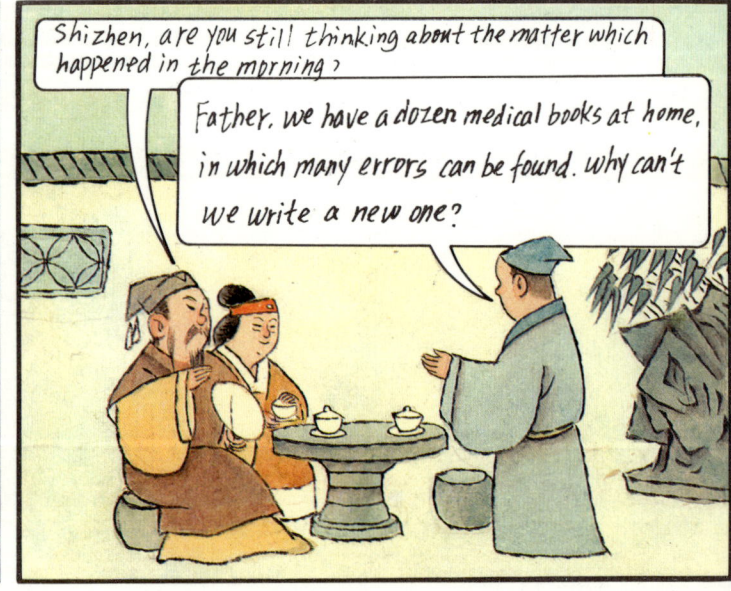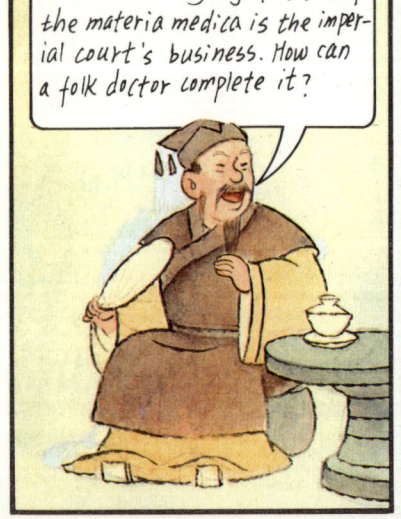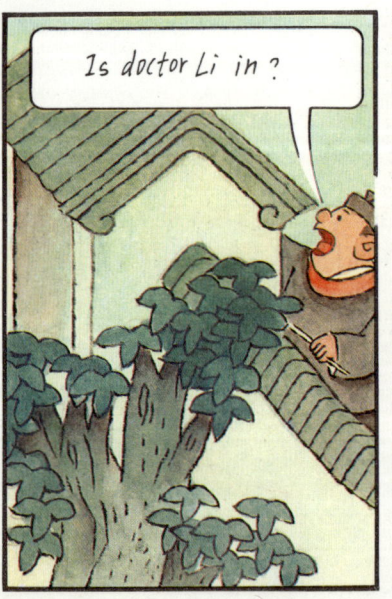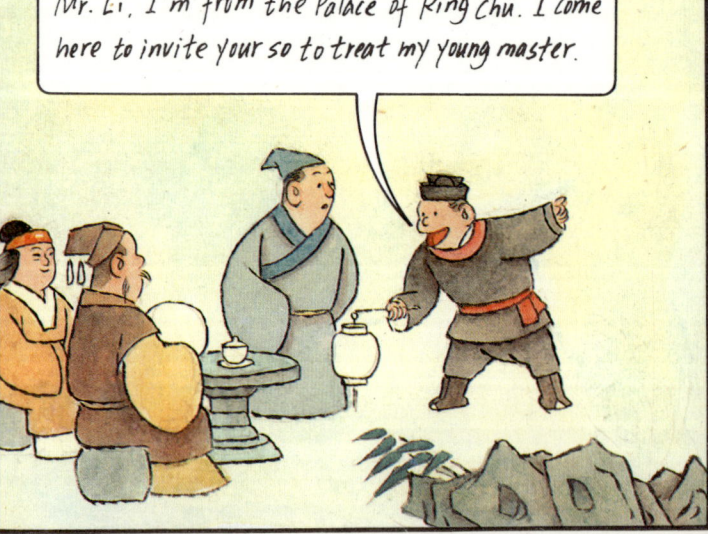

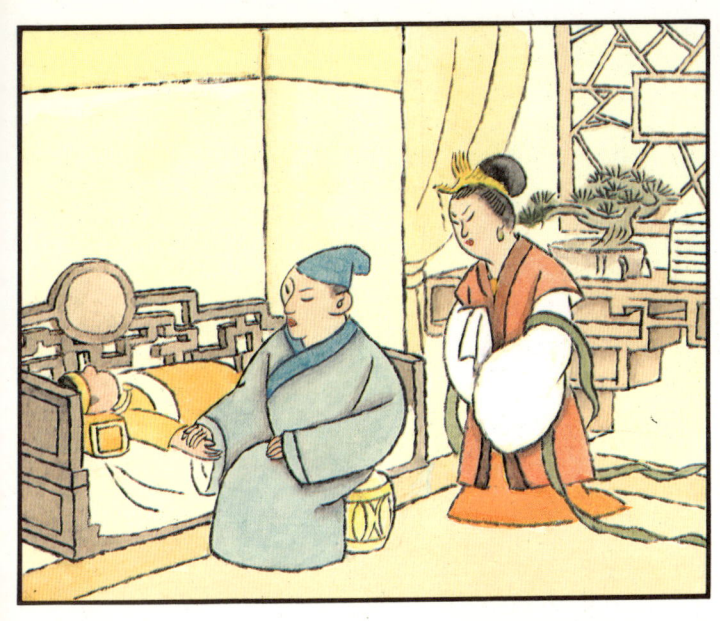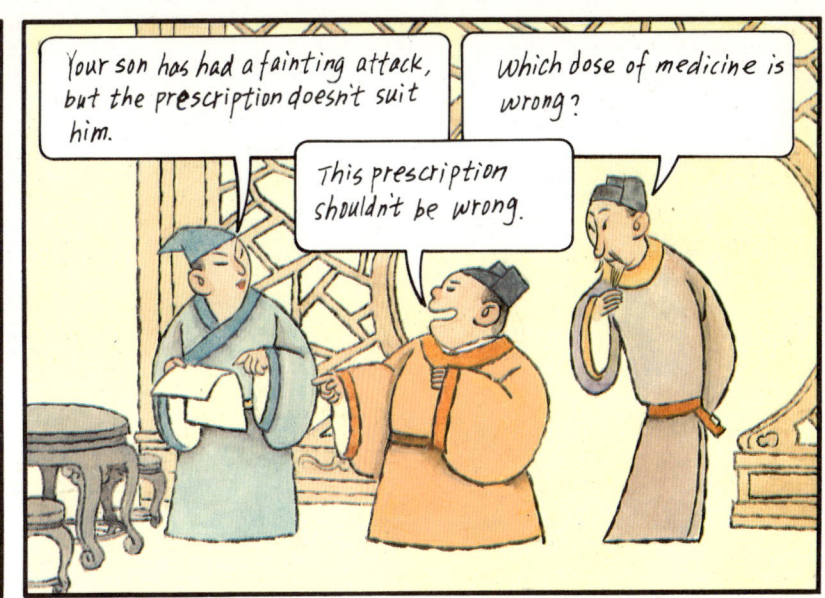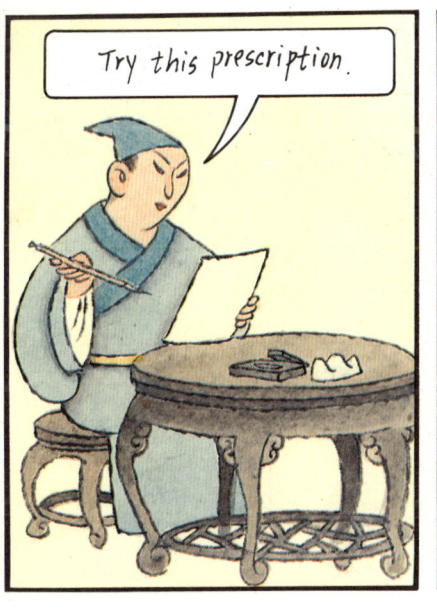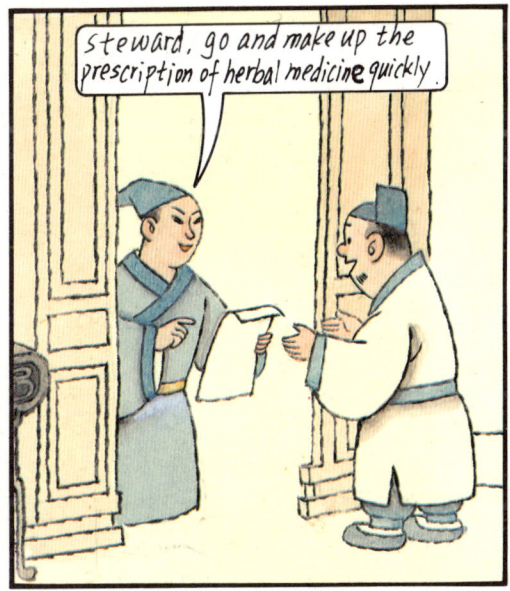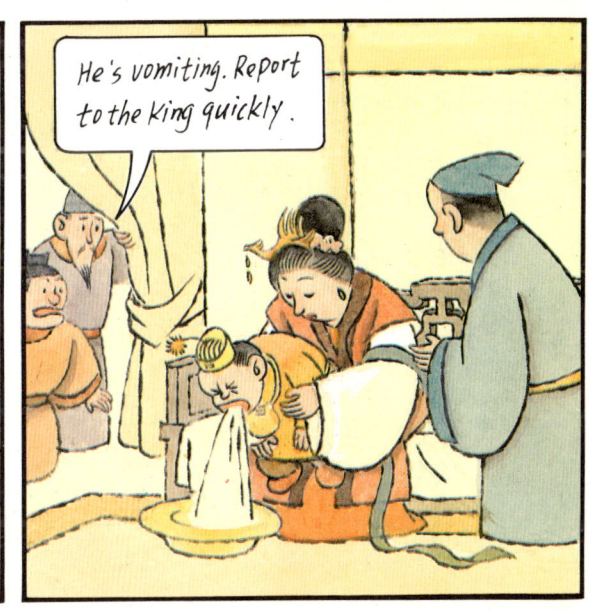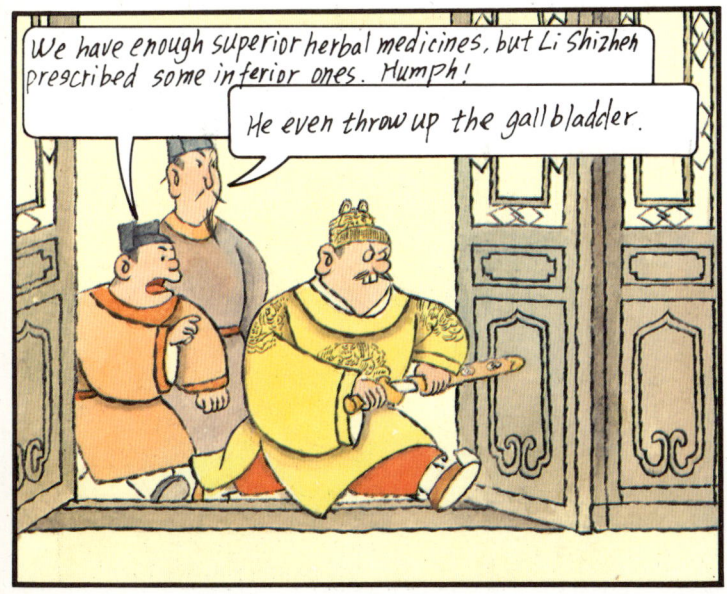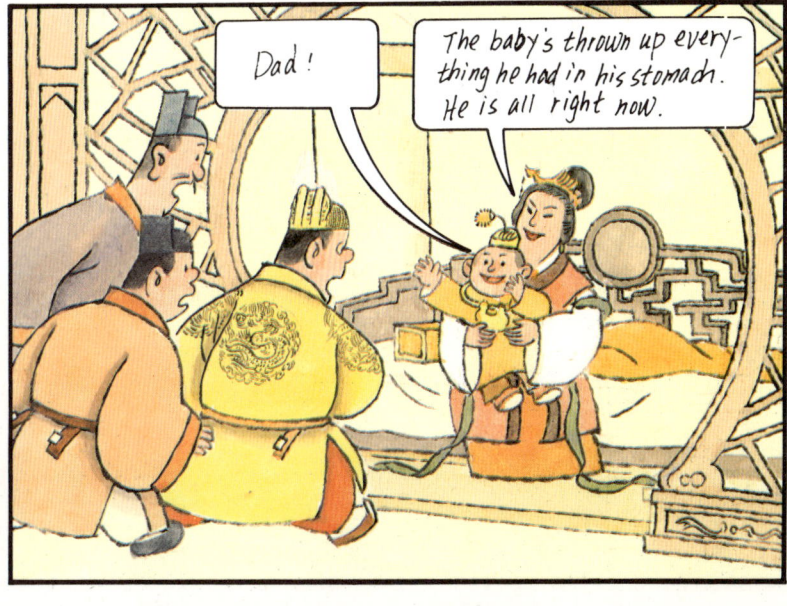

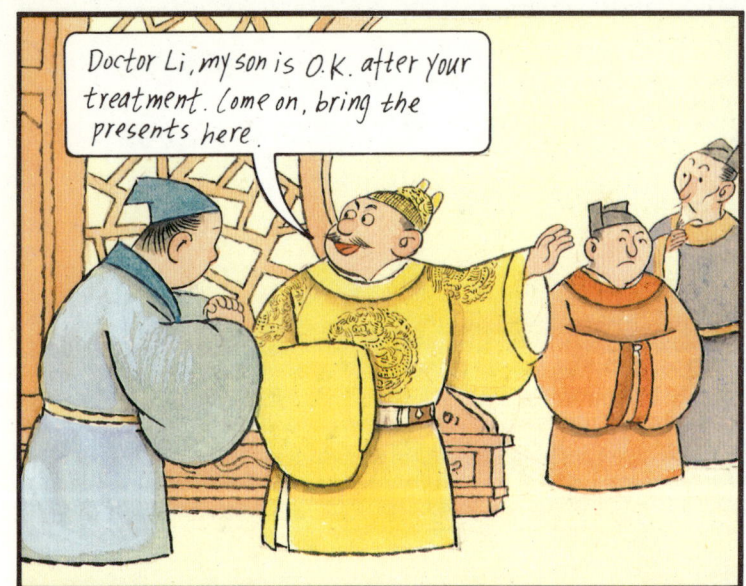

"Doctor Li, my son is O.K. after your treatment. Come on, bring the presents here."

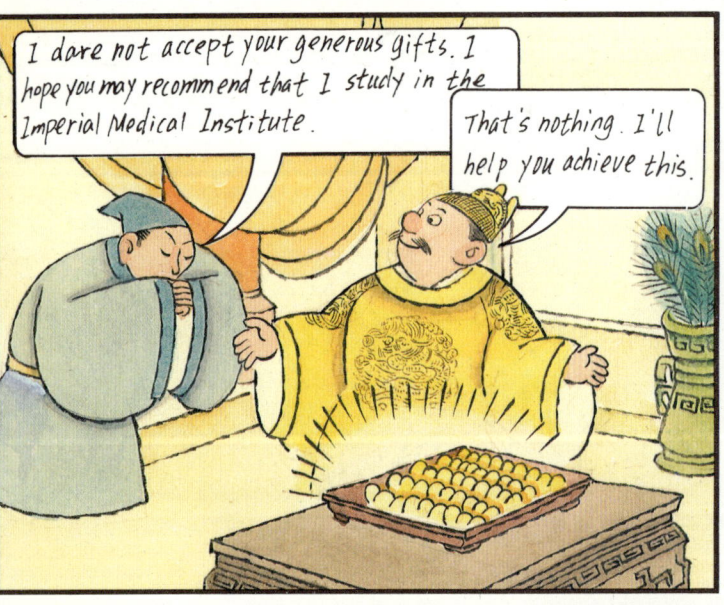

"I dare not accept your generous gifts. I hope you may recommend that I study in the Imperial Medical Institute."

"That's nothing. I'll help you achieve this."

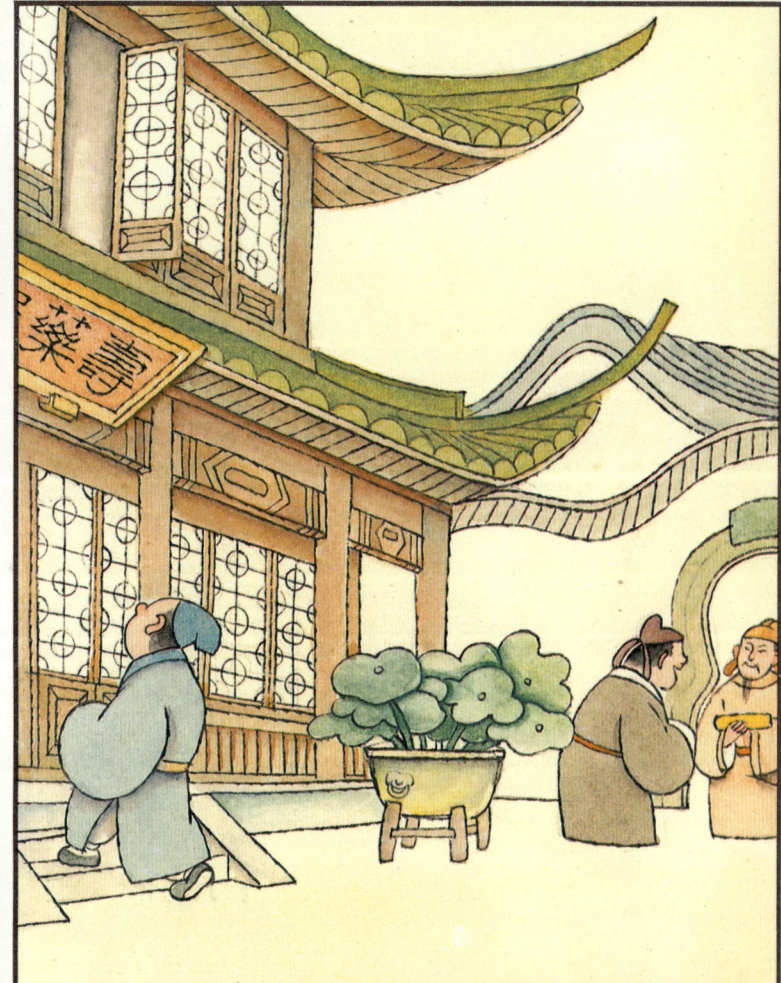

In 1556, Li Shizhen was appointed chief director of the Imperial Medical Institute. Usually he did not have much to do, so he stayed in the House of Longevity Medicine, and the Storehouse of Imperial Medicine, gaining knowledge about all sorts of herbal medicines.

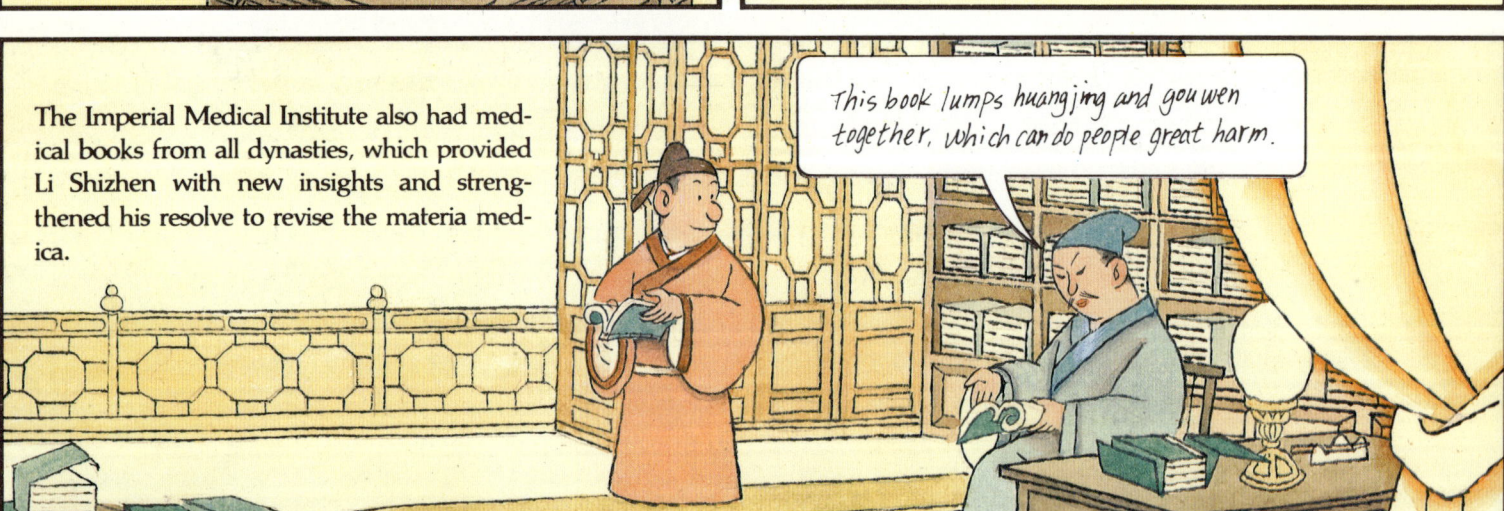

The Imperial Medical Institute also had medical books from all dynasties, which provided Li Shizhen with new insights and strengthened his resolve to revise the materia medica.

"This book lumps huangjing and gouwen together, which can do people great harm."

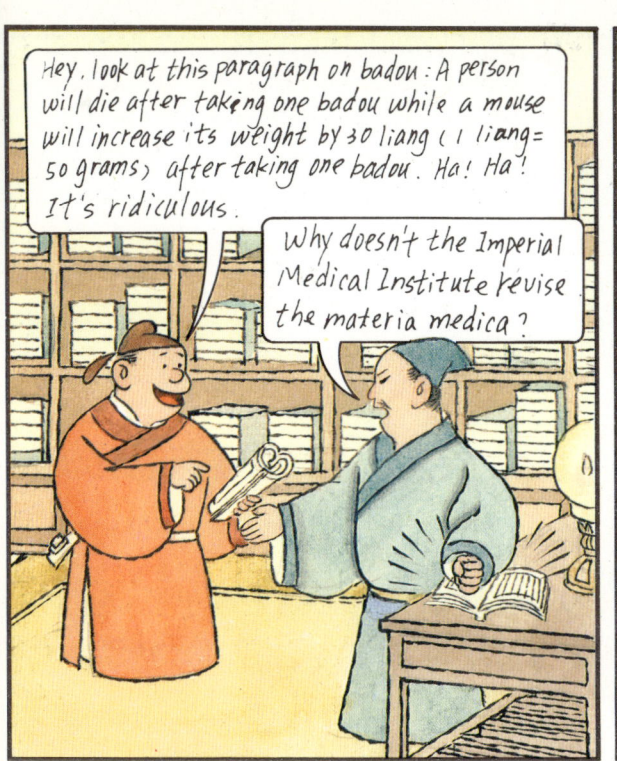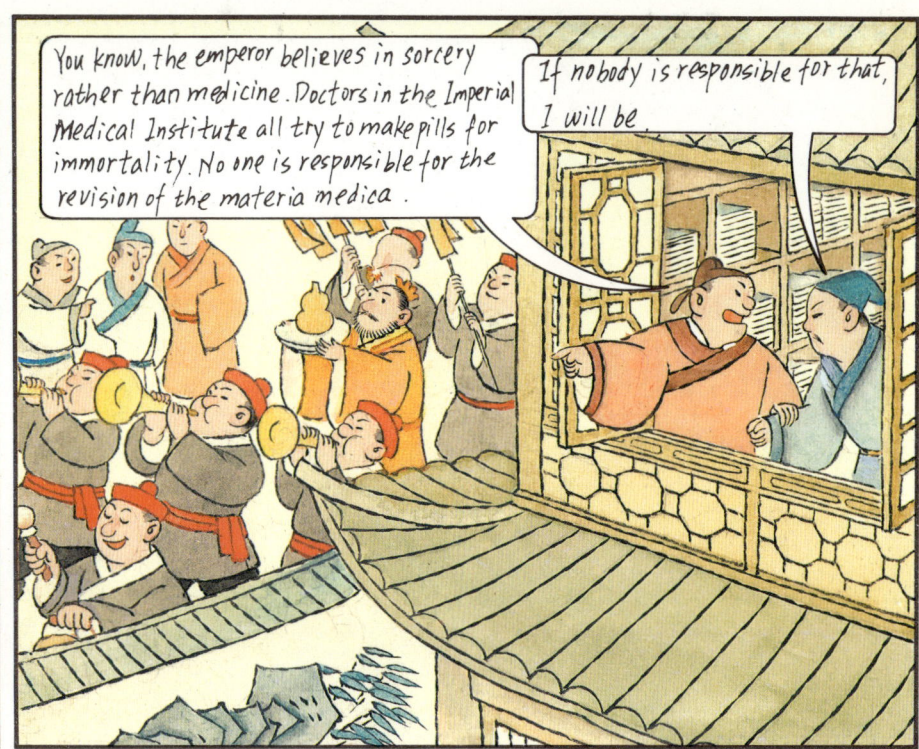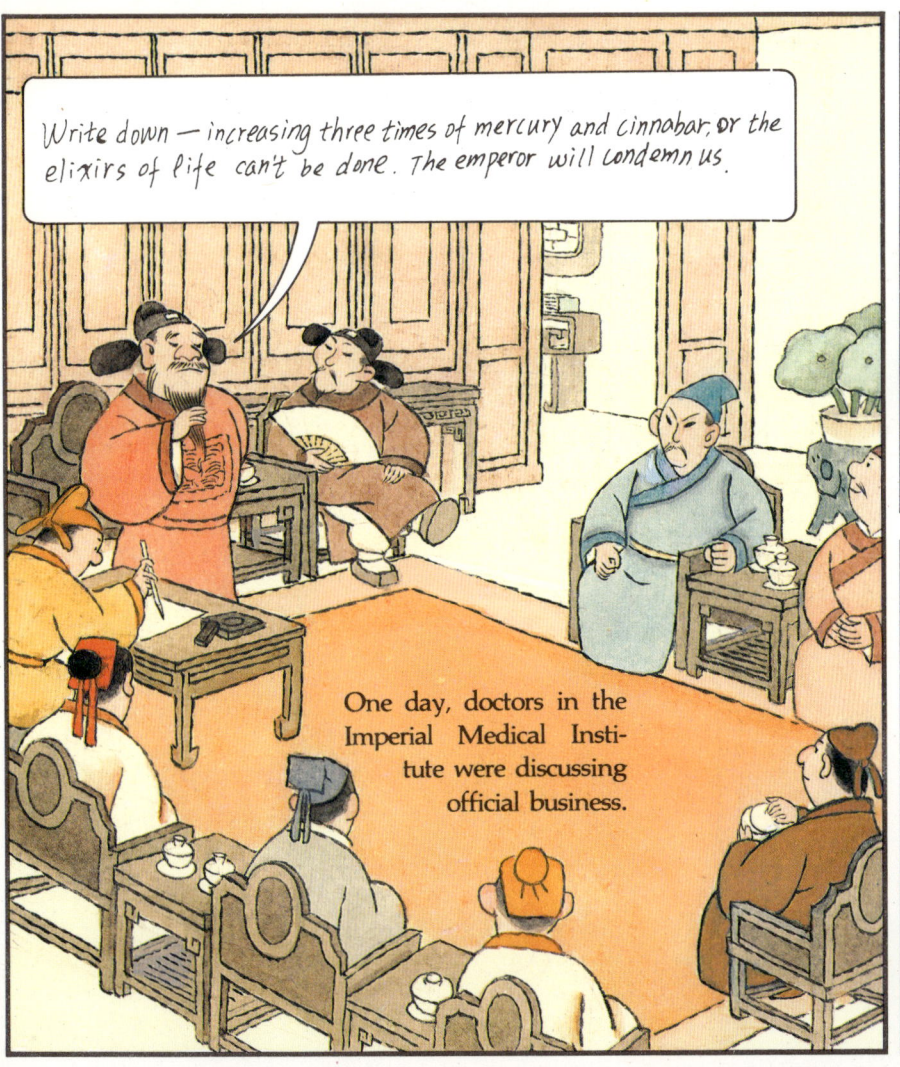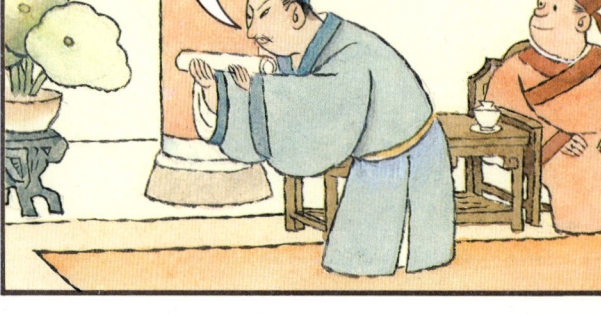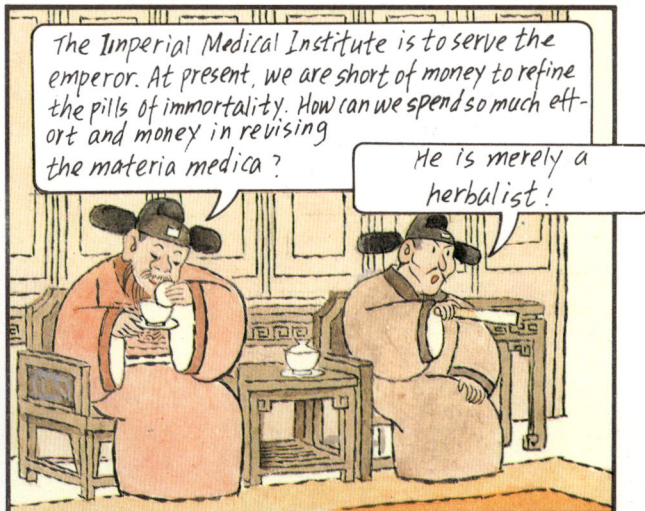

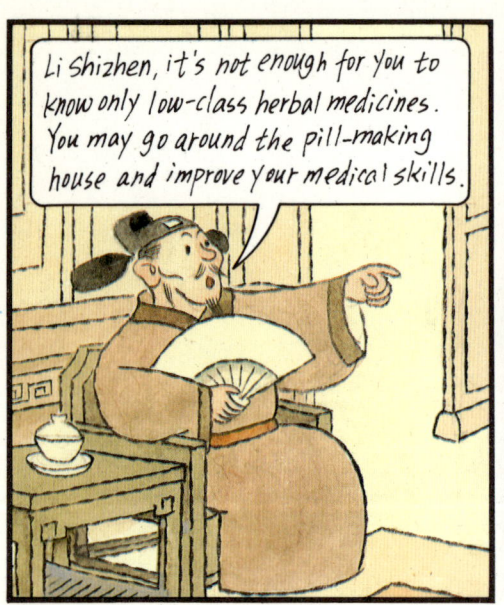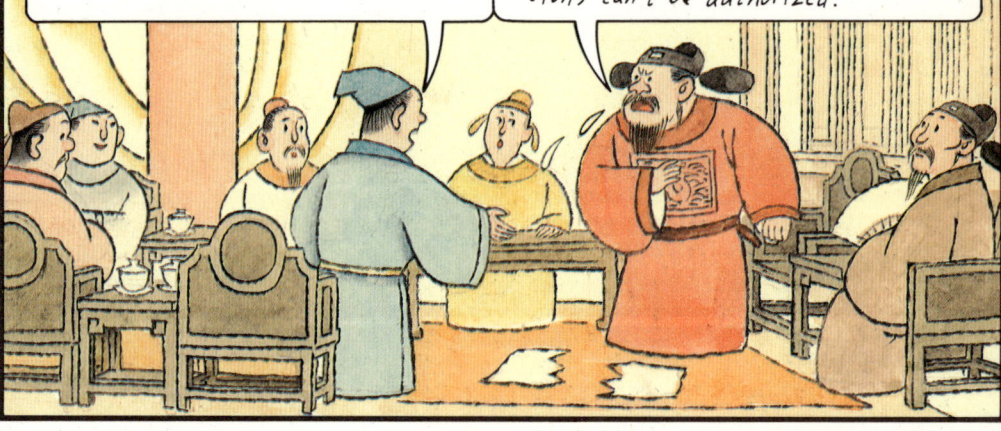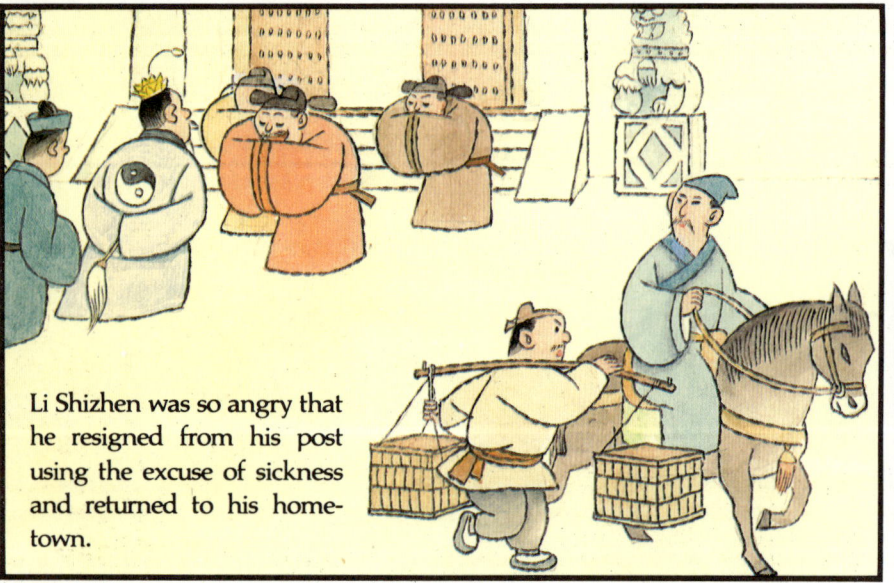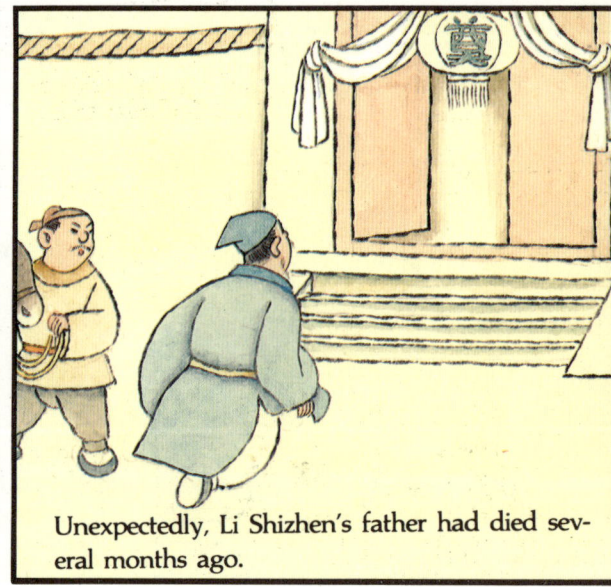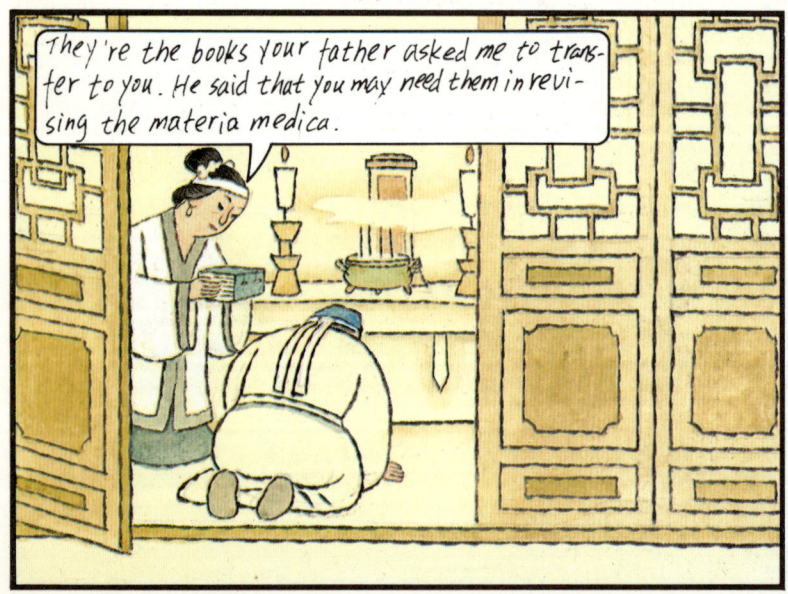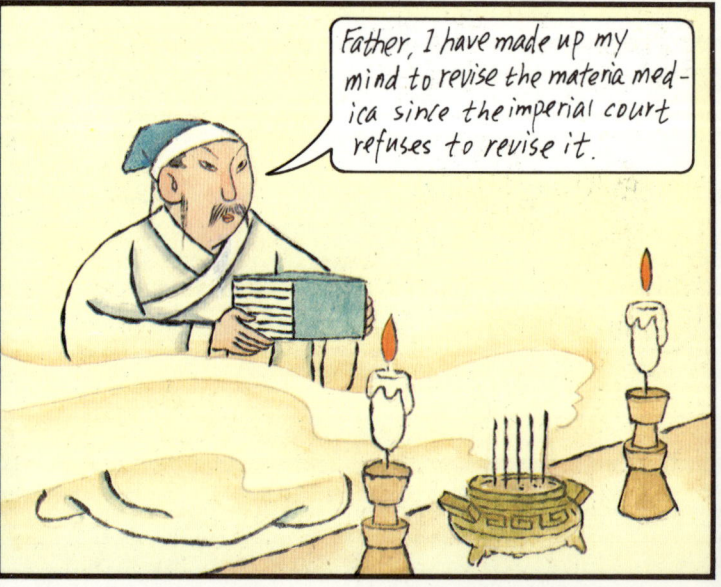

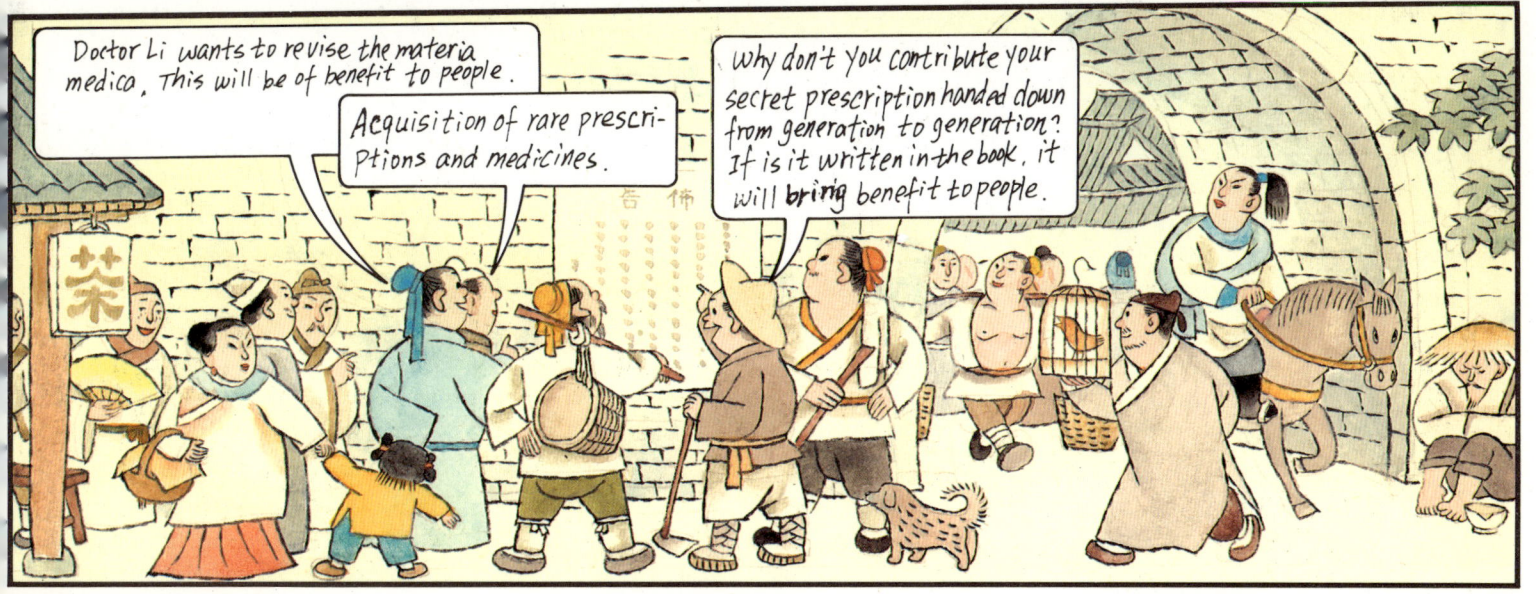
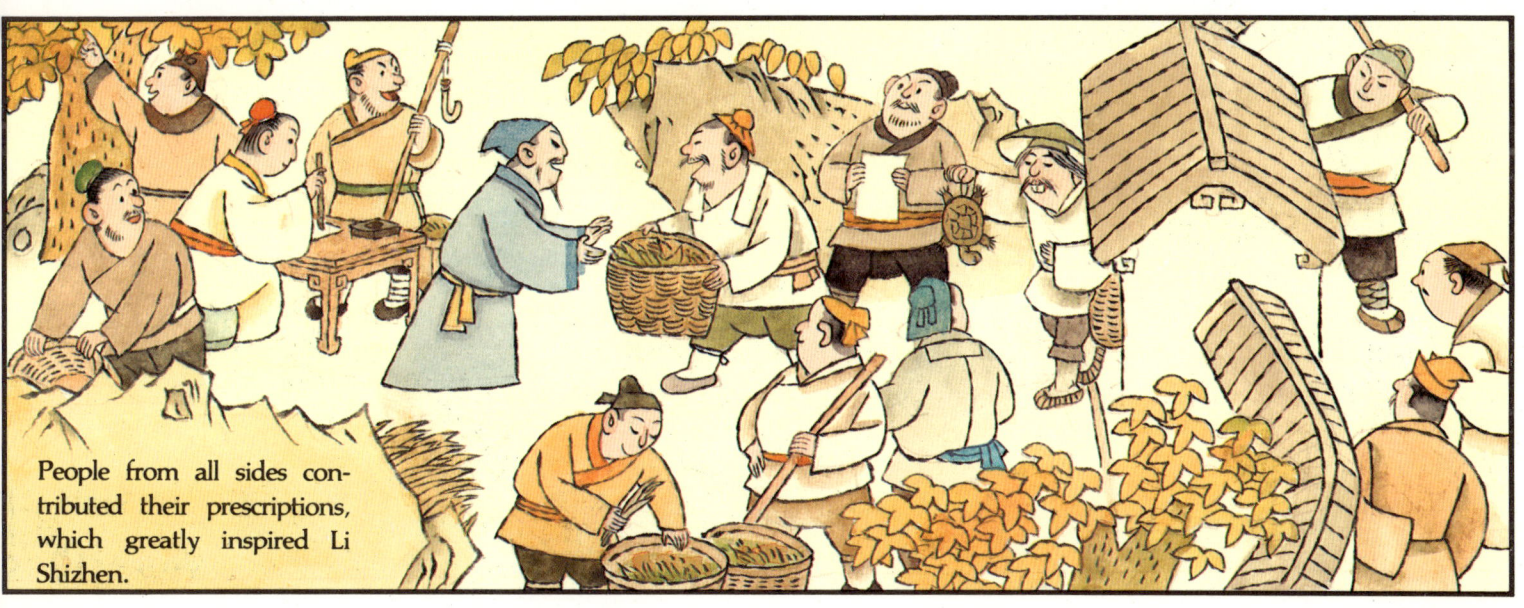
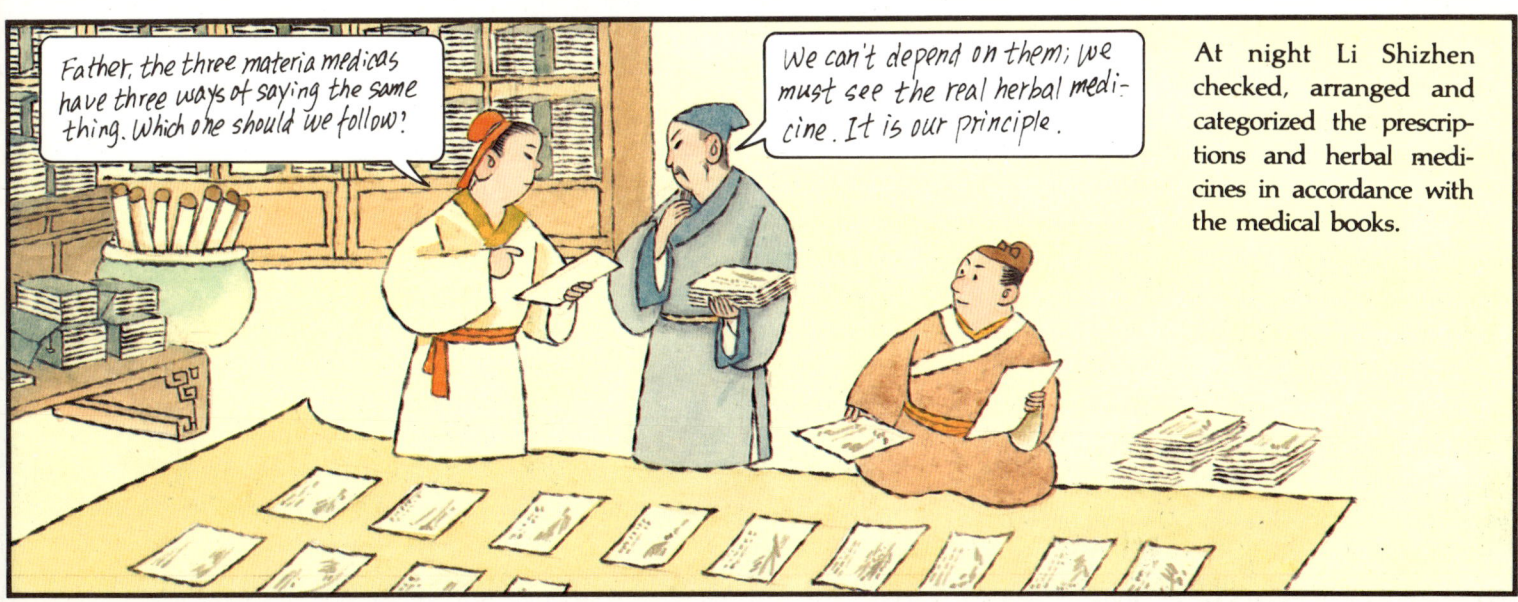

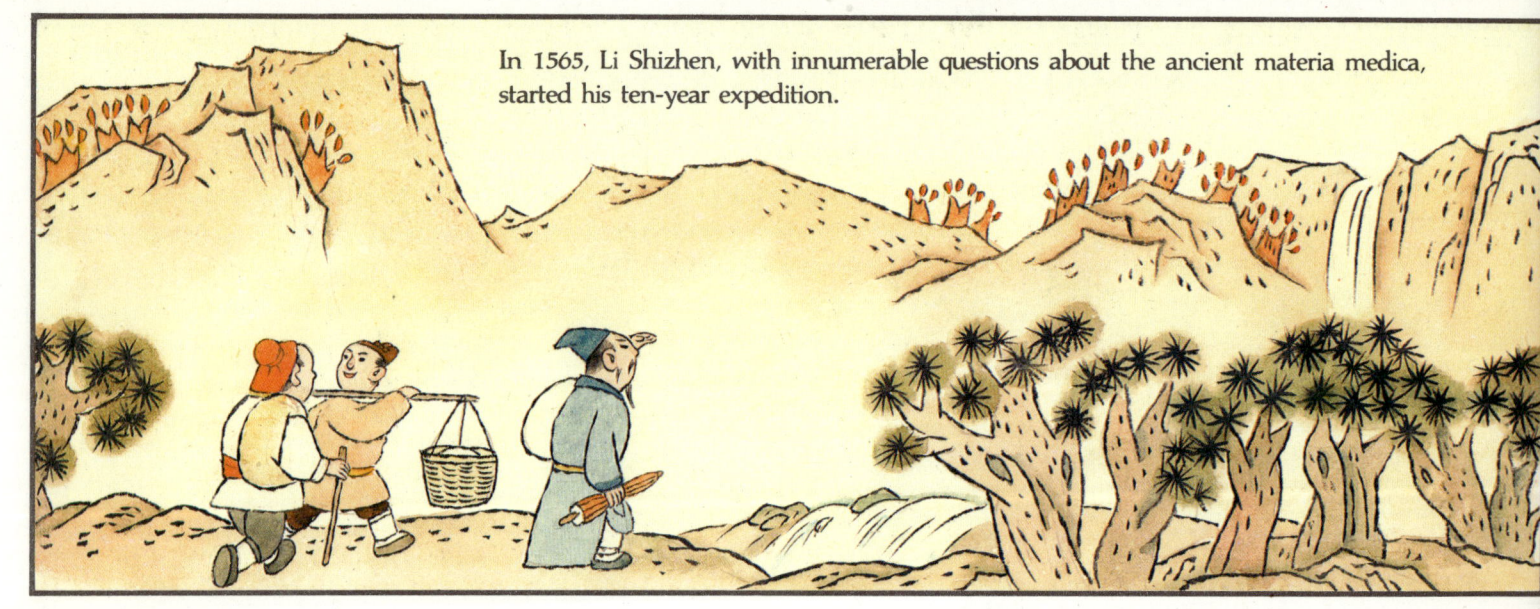

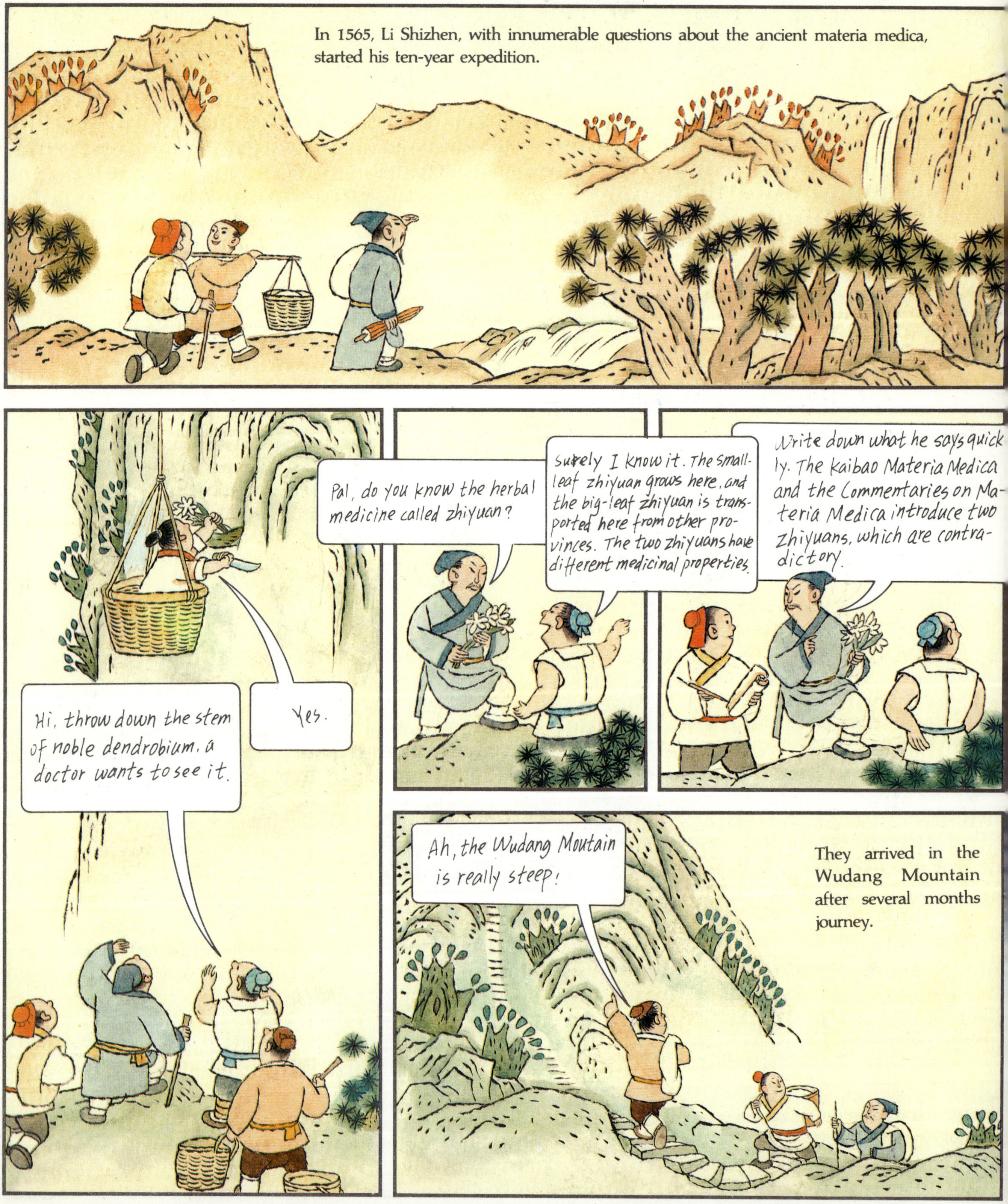

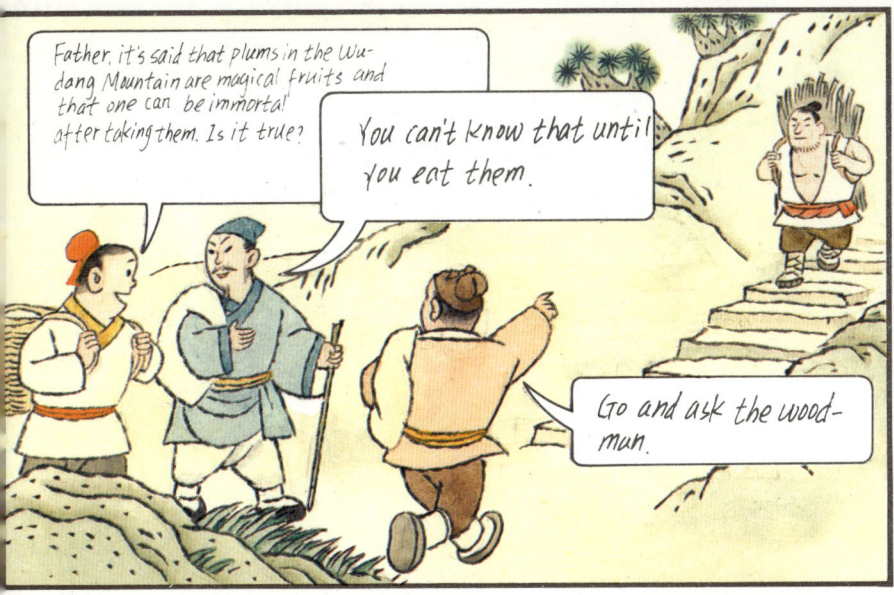
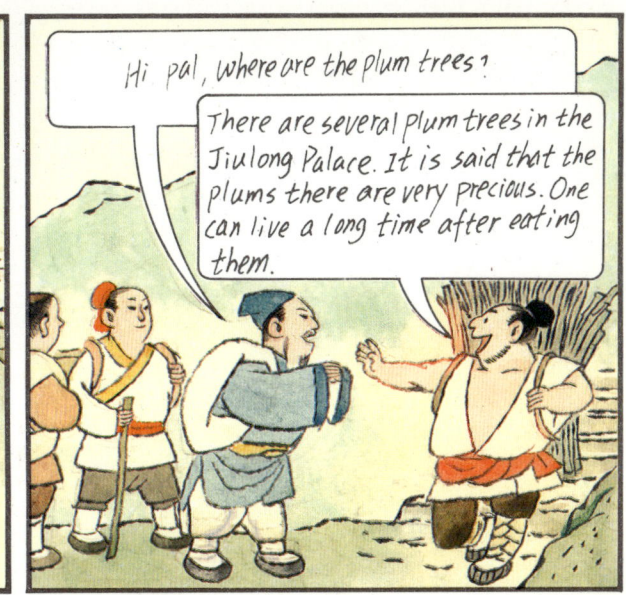
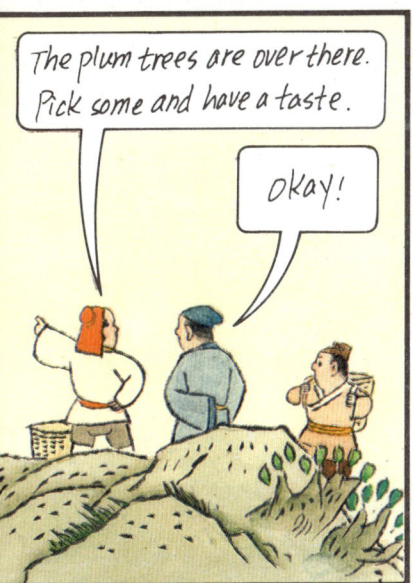
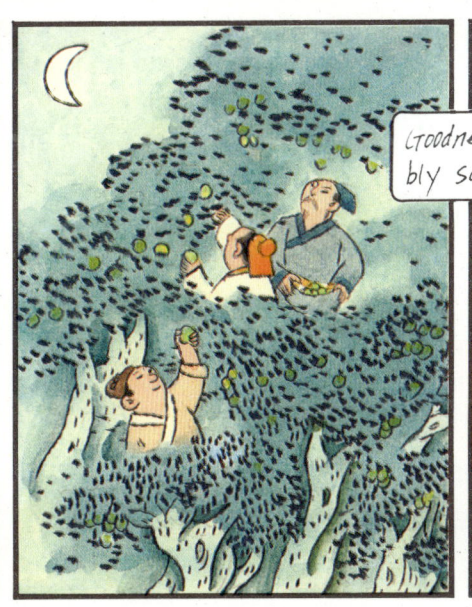
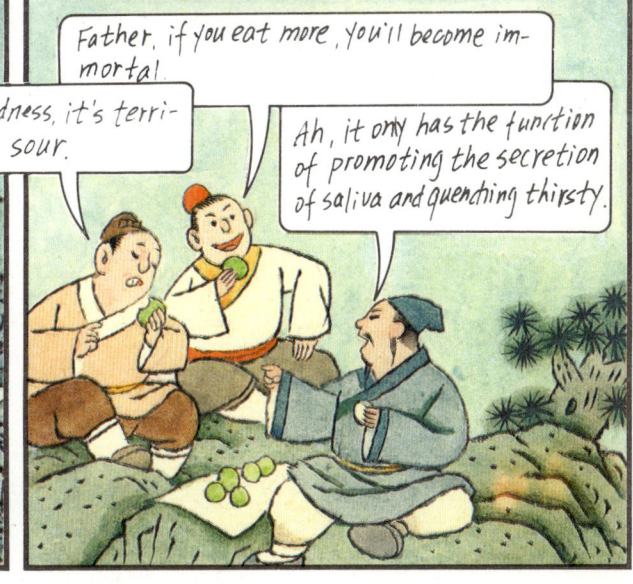
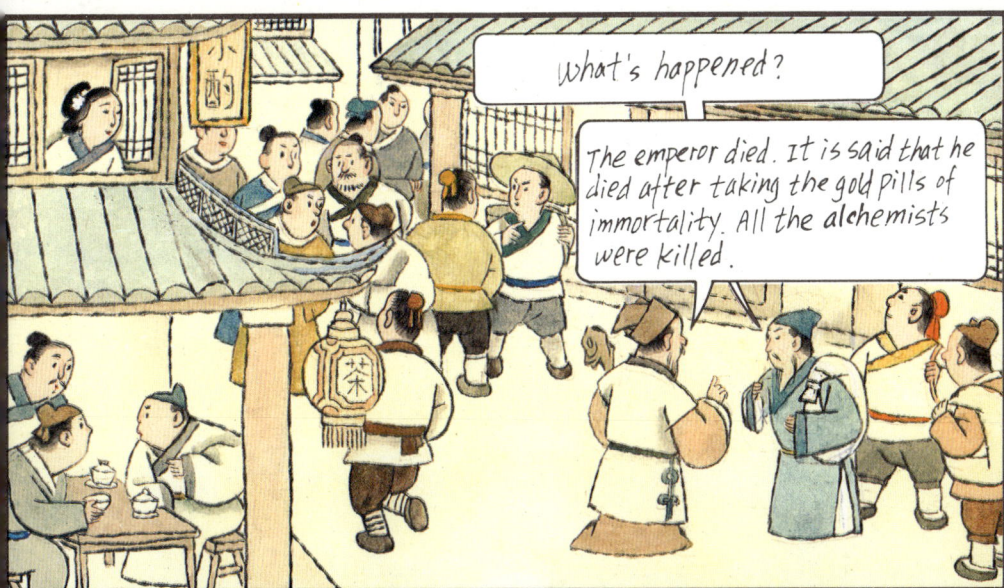
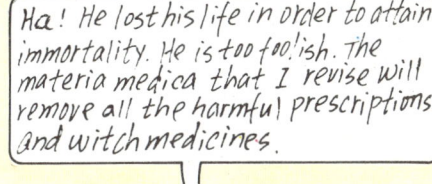
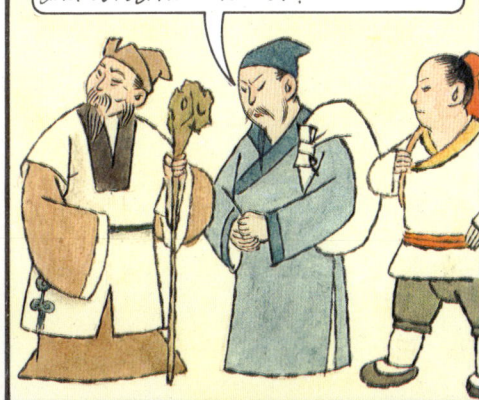

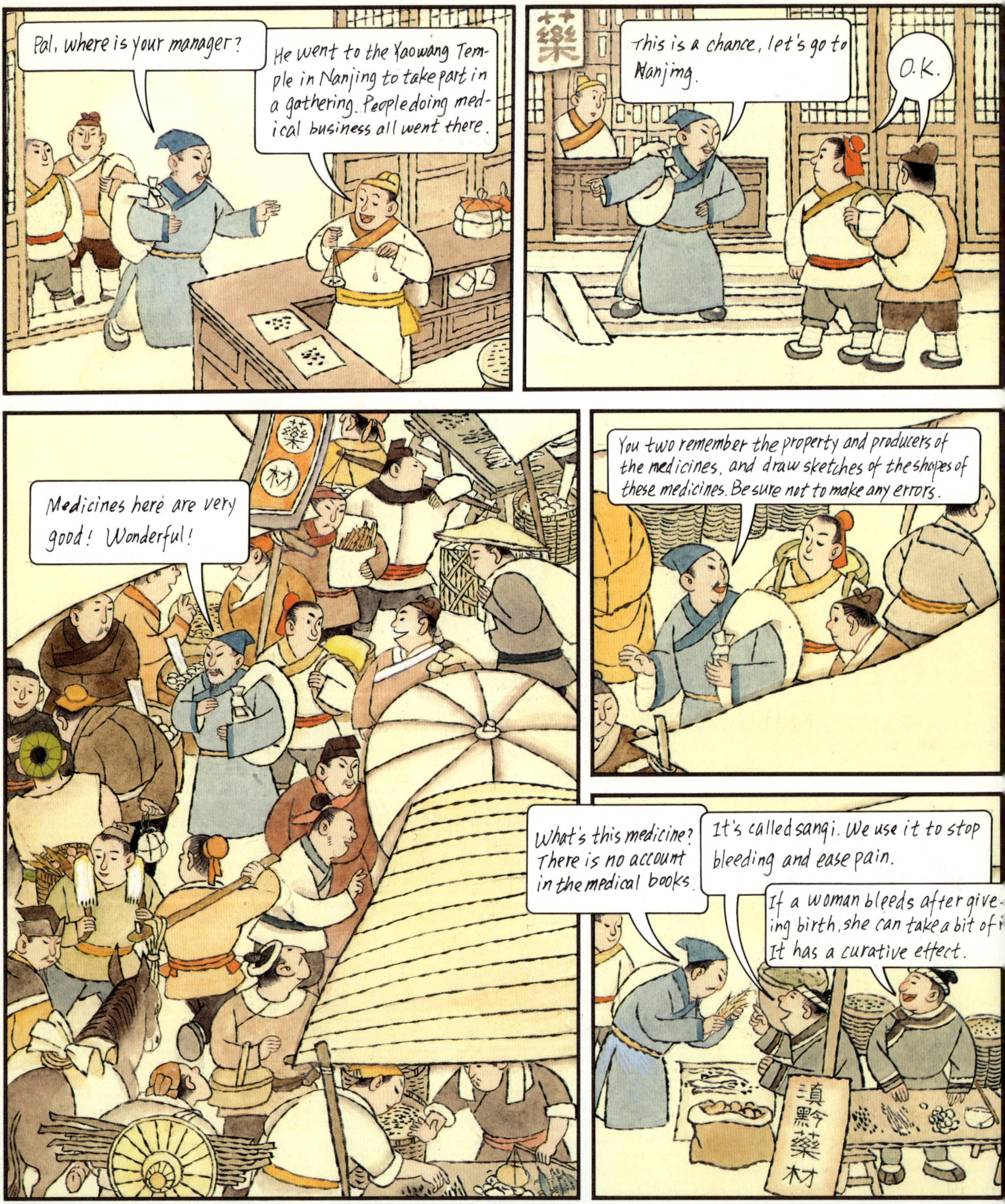

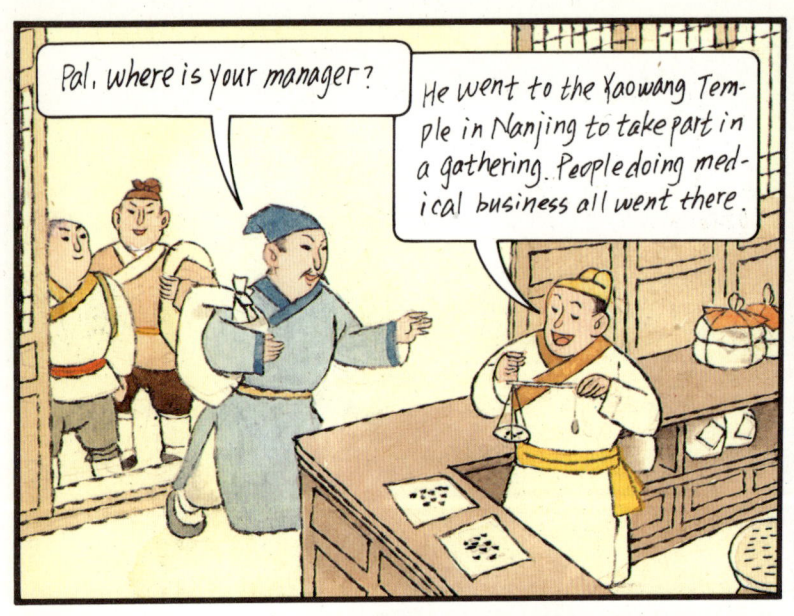
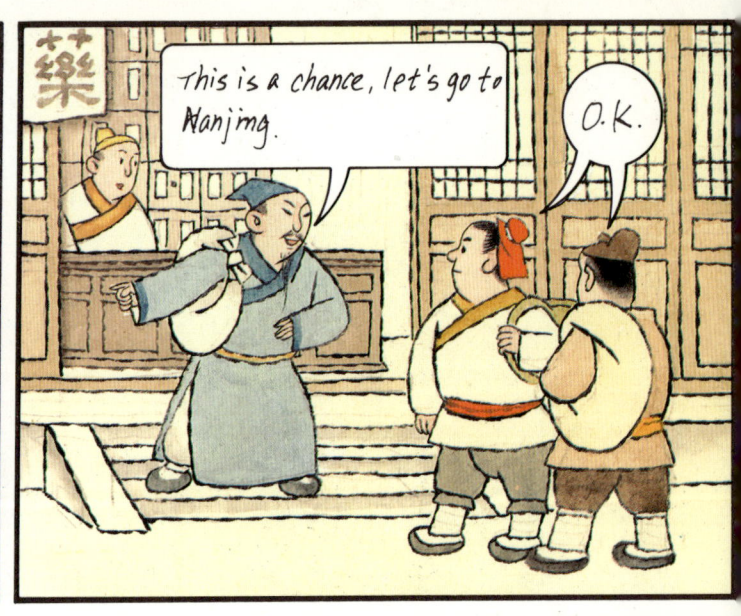
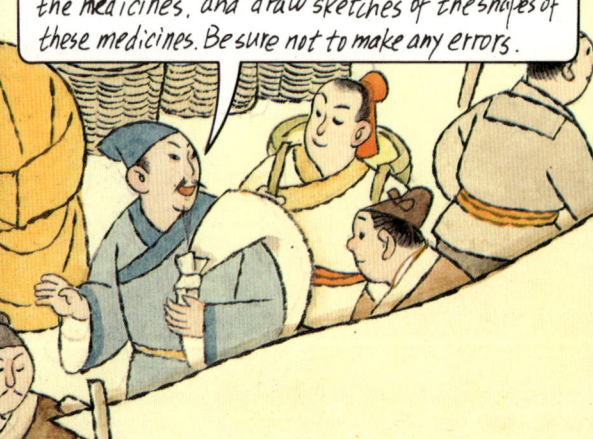

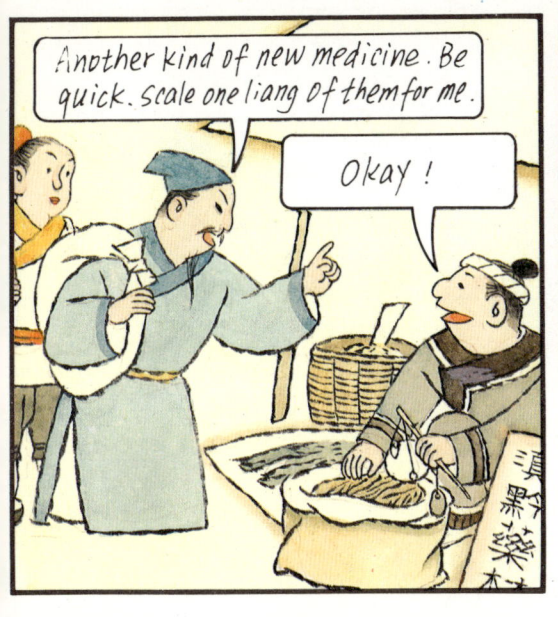
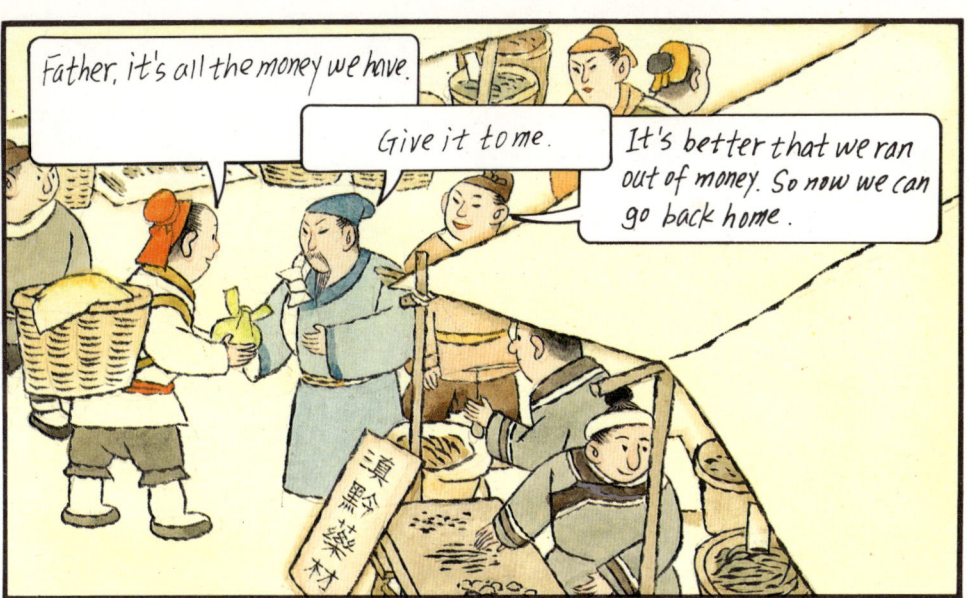
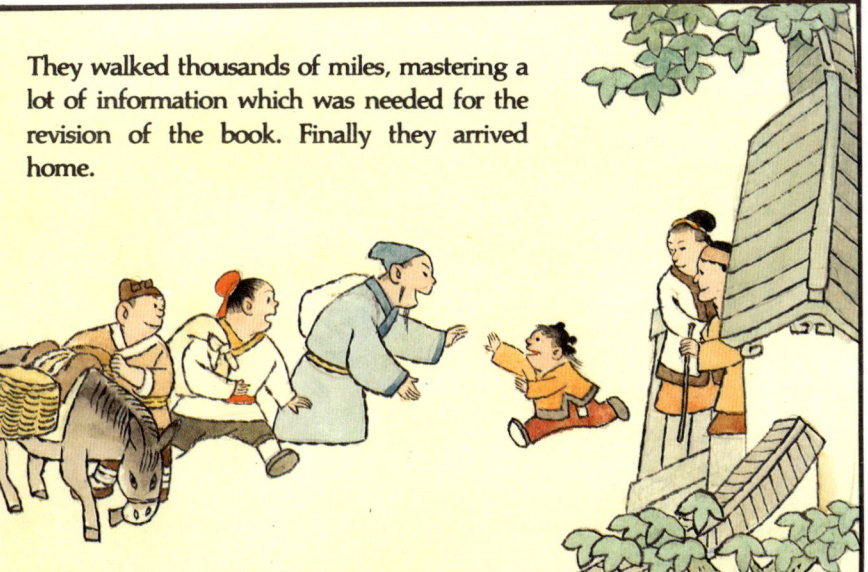
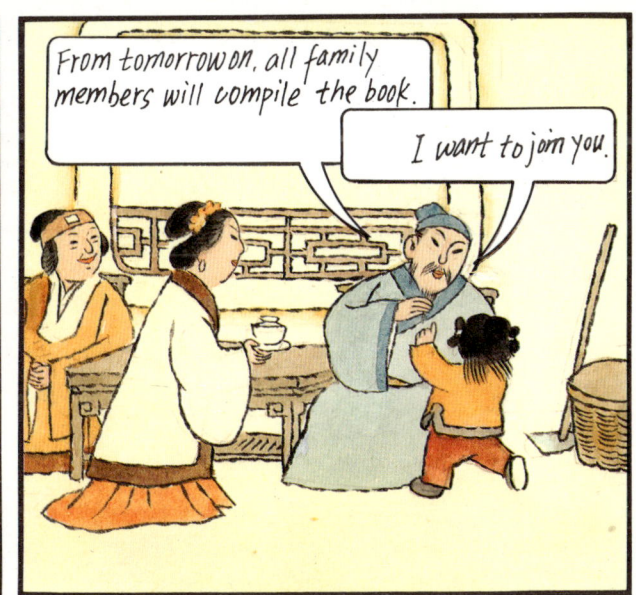
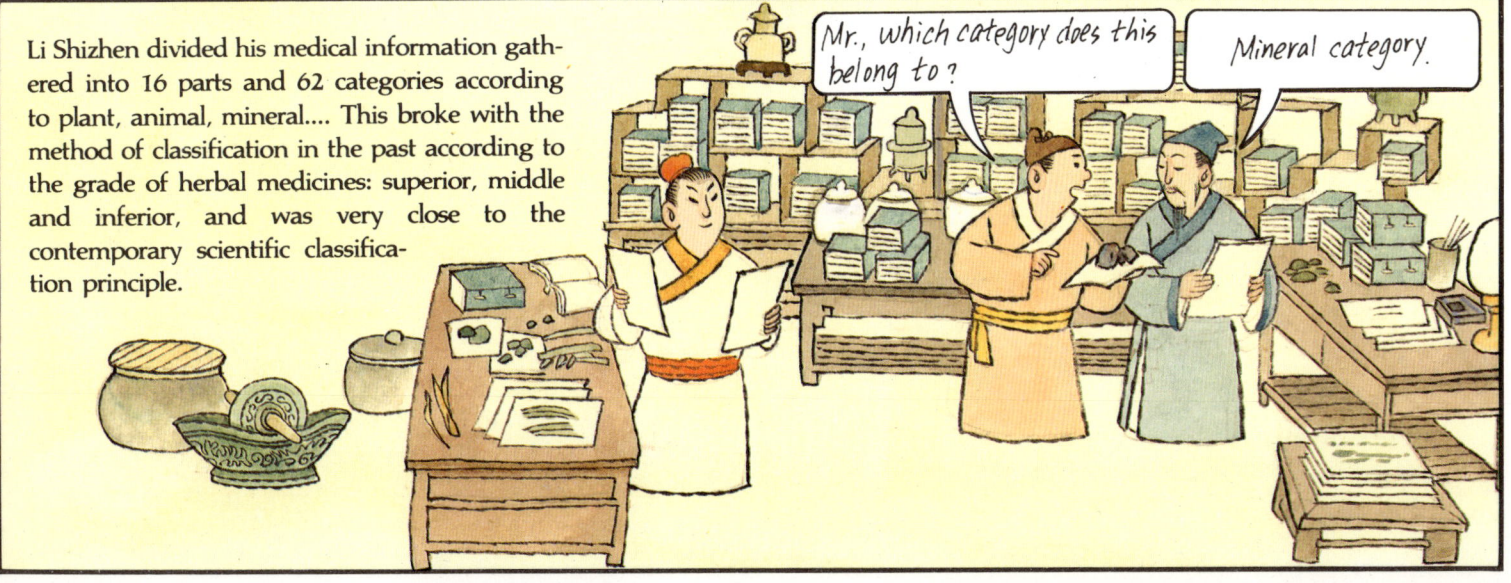

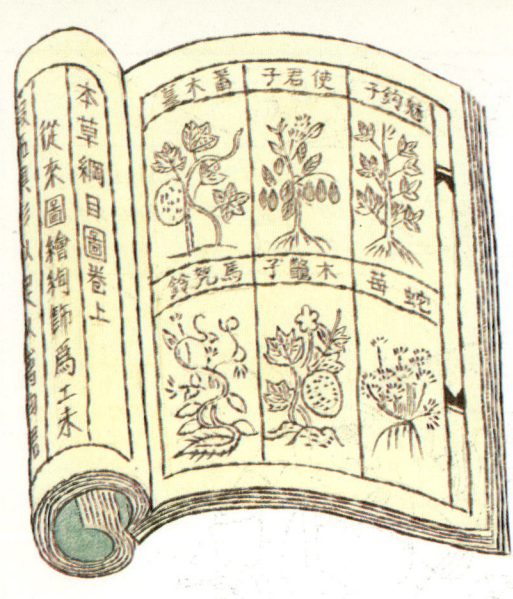

Li Shizhen wrote down in detail the name, producing area, shape, cultivating and collecting method, smell and function of each medicine, and enclosed the shape sketch of each medicine.

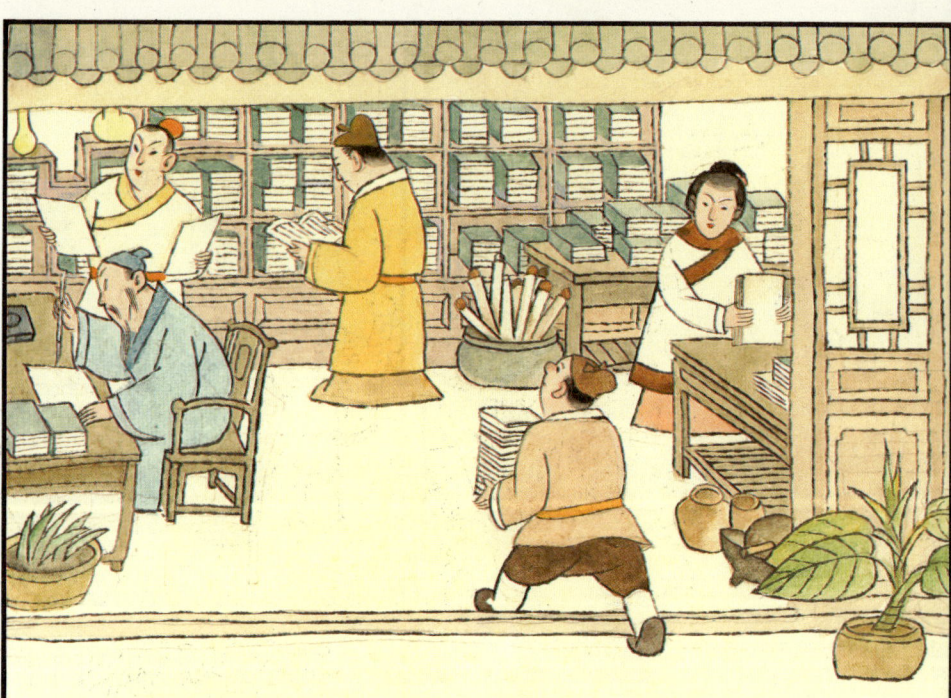

After 27 years of hard work, at the age of 61, Li Shizhen finally completed the monumental work entitled the *Compendium of Materia Medica*.

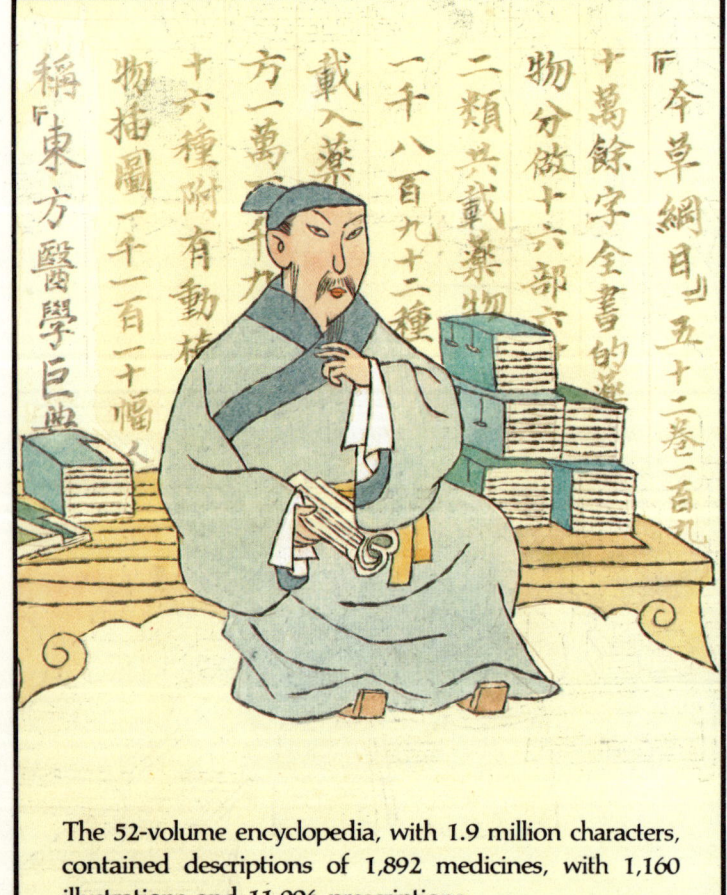

The 52-volume encyclopedia, with 1.9 million characters, contained descriptions of 1,892 medicines, with 1,160 illustrations and 11,096 prescriptions.

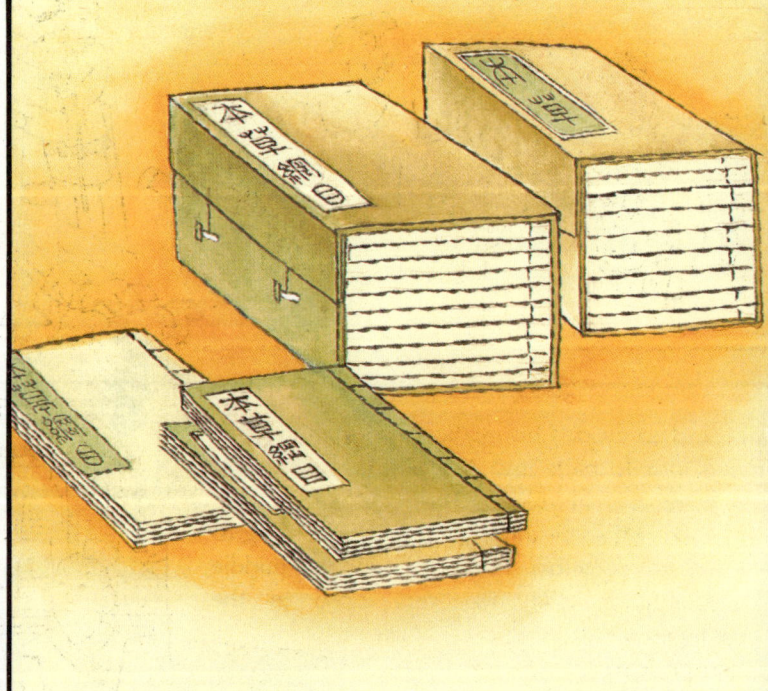

In 1596, the *Compendium of Materia Medica* came out, causing a great stir. Bookstores all over the country made copies of the book one after another. It became a great classic work of Chinese medicine. By then, Li Shizhen had been dead for three years. Later, the book reputed as the great medical work in the Orient was translated into many languages.